ABC of
Stroke

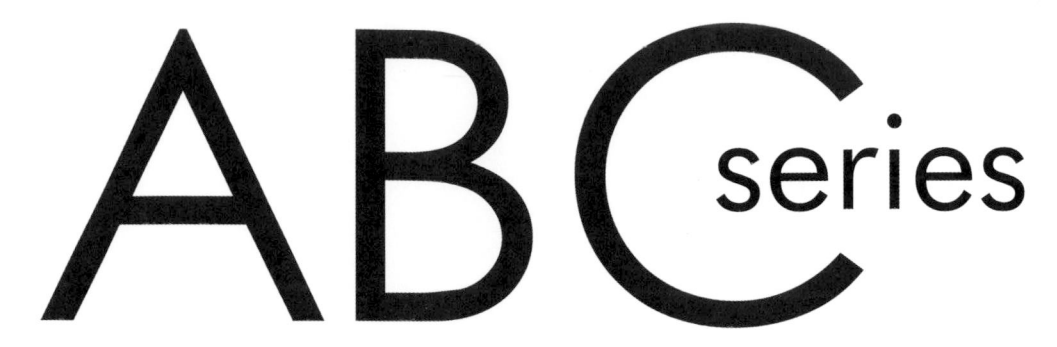
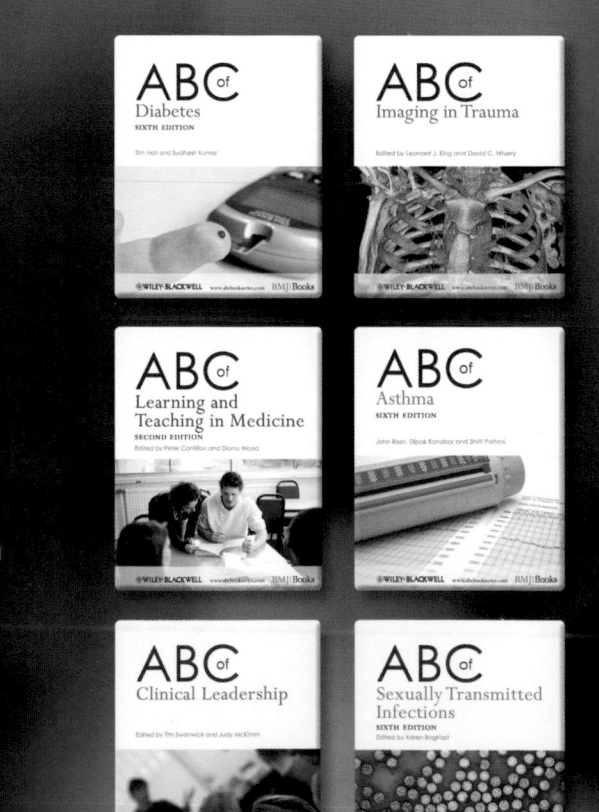

ABC of
Stroke

EDITED BY

Jonathan Mant

Associate Director UK Stroke Research Network *and*
Professor of Primary Care Research
Addenbrooke's Hospital, University of Cambridge, UK

Marion F Walker

Associate Director UK Stroke Research Network *and*
Professor in Stroke Rehabilitation
University of Nottingham, UK

WILEY-BLACKWELL
A John Wiley & Sons, Ltd., Publication

BMJ | Books

Library of Congress Cataloging-in-Publication Data

ABC of stroke / edited by Jonathan Mant, Associate Director, UK Stroke Research Network and Professor of Primary Care Research, Addenbrookes Hospital, University of Cambridge, UK, Marion F. Walker, Associate Director, UK Stroke Research Network and Professor in Stroke Rehabilitation, University of Nottingham, UK.

p. ; cm.
Includes bibliographical references and index.
ISBN 978-1-4051-6790-1 (pbk. : alk. paper) 1. Cerebrovascular disease. I. Mant, J. (Jonathan), editor. II. Walker, Marion F., editor.
[DNLM: 1. Stroke. WL 355]
RC388.5.A23 2011
616.8′1 – dc22

2010047394

This book is published in the following electronic formats: ePDF 9781444397789; ePub 9781444397796

A catalogue record for this book is available from the British Library.

Set in 9.25/12 Minion by Laserwords Private Limited, Chennai, India
Printed and bound in Malaysia by Vivar Printing Sdn Bhd

1   2011

Contents

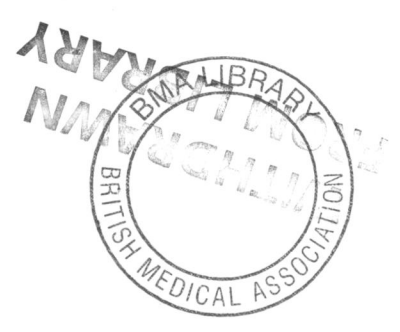

Contributors

Jane Barton

Consultant Clinical Psychologist, Sheffield Health and Social Care Foundation, NHS Trust, Sheffield, UK

Duncan Edwards

Academic Clinical Fellow in General Practice, University of Cambridge, Cambridge, UK

Pam Enderby

Professor of Community Rehabilitation, School of Health and Related Research, University of Sheffield, Sheffield, UK

Clare Gordon

Nurse Consultant in Stroke, Stroke Unit, The Royal Bournemouth and Christchurch Hospitals' NHS Trust, Christchurch, UK

Damian Jenkinson

Clinical Director, Stroke Unit, The Royal Bournemouth and Christchurch Hospitals' NHS Trust, Christchurch, UK

Jonathan Mant

Associate Director UK Stroke Research Network and Professor of Primary Care Research, General Practice & Primary Care Research Unit, Department of Public Health & Primary Care, Addenbrooke's Hospital, University of Cambridge, Cambridge, UK

Marion F Walker

Associate Director UK Stroke Research Network and Professor in Stroke Rehabilitation, School of Community Health Sciences, Faculty of Medicine & Health Science, University of Nottingham, Nottingham, UK

Preface

Stroke is one of the top three causes of death and the largest cause of adult disability in England, and costs the NHS over £3 billion a year.

– National Audit Office 2010

Over 100 000 people have a stroke in England each year and come into contact with a wide range of health-care professionals, each with their own area of expertise. There are many excellent textbooks that focus on these individual specialties. What we felt was needed was a book that provided an overview of the multi-faceted aspects of stroke care: a book that would provide a useful summary for the specialist of those aspects of stroke care in which they were not directly involved, and a guide for the generalist to the range of services and treatments that are available. Indeed, in the longer term, much of the contact of people with stroke will be with members of the primary care team, such as the general practitioner and practice nurse, and few previous books about stroke have addressed the needs of this target audience. We also hope the book will appeal to people with stroke and their families – surveys continue to show that lack of information remains a major problem. If this book can go a small way to addressing this, then it will have been worth writing.

Stroke has had a much lower profile than heart disease and cancer. This is changing, however. There is a growing public awareness of stroke, and we hope to contribute to this increasing knowledge through the *ABC of Stroke*. Our aim has been to cover both the medical and the non-medical aspects of stroke, and to give as much weight to the longer-term community aspects of care as to the acute hospital-based components of care, which can tend to dominate traditional medical textbooks.

We hope that the *ABC of Stroke* will provide readers with an accessible overview of the problems faced by people with stroke and their carers and possible ways in which they can be addressed.

Jonathan Mant,
University of Cambridge

Marion Walker,
University of Nottingham

CHAPTER 1

Introduction to Stroke

Jonathan Mant

Addenbrooke's Hospital, University of Cambridge, UK

OVERVIEW

- Stroke is a syndrome of sudden onset of neurological symptoms, which may be either ischaemic or haemorrhagic in origin
- Stroke is the commonest cause of adult disability
- Age-specific stroke incidence and mortality are falling, but overall incidence may increase in the future due to population ageing
- Key risk factors for stroke are hypertension, smoking and atrial fibrillation
- Maximal physical recovery is usually seen within six months of stroke, but recovery of more complex abilities (e.g. speech) may continue over years

---

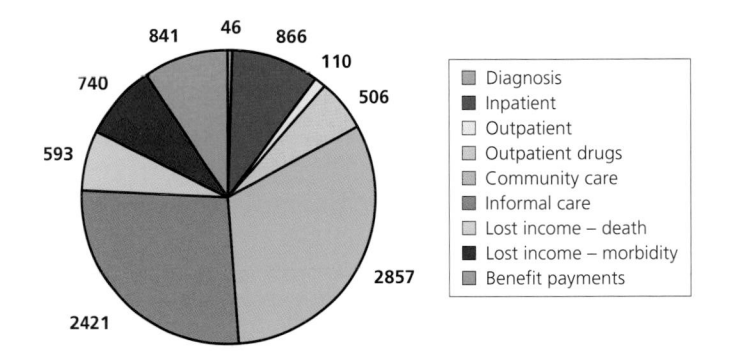

Figure 1.1 Costs of stroke care (numbers represent £m). *Source*: Saka O, McGuire A, Wolfe C. Cost of stroke in the United Kingdom. *Age and Ageing* 2009;**38**:27–32.

A stroke is a sudden onset of neurological impairment that is caused by a disruption of the blood supply to the brain (see Box 1.1). If the duration of the impairment is less than 24 hours, the event is referred to as a transient ischaemic attack (TIA) rather than a stroke; see Chapter 3. There are two main types of stroke: ischaemic stroke, and haemorrhagic stroke. Ischaemic stroke is caused by obstruction of a blood vessel supplying the brain, either due to in-situ thrombus or embolus from a distant site (most commonly the carotid arteries or the heart). Haemorrhagic stroke is caused by bleeding of a blood vessel supplying the brain. Subarachnoid haemorrhage, which usually occurs as a result of rupturing of an aneurysm, may also lead to stroke, but the clinical features and management are very different from stroke and are not covered in this book.

Box 1.1 **A definition of stroke**

Stroke is a clinical syndrome characterised by an acute loss of focal cerebral function with symptoms lasting more than 24 hours or leading to death, and which is thought to be due to either spontaneous haemorrhage into the brain substance (haemorrhagic stroke) or inadequate cerebral blood supply to a part of the brain (ischaemic stroke) as a result of low blood flow, thrombosis or embolism associated with diseases of the blood vessels (arteries or veins), heart or blood.

Source: Warlow C, van Gijn J, Dennis M *et al. Stroke: Practical Management*. 3rd edn, Ch 3. Oxford: Blackwell Publishing, 2008, pp.35–130

ABC of Stroke. Edited by Jonathan Mant and Marion F Walker.
© 2011 Blackwell Publishing Ltd.

Stroke accounted for over 46 000 deaths (9% of all deaths) in England and Wales in 2008, and it is the commonest cause of adult disability, with about 300 000 people in England living with moderate to severe disability as a result of stroke. The total cost to the UK of stroke, taking into account the costs of informal care and of lost income, are around £9 billion per year (Figure 1.1). Inpatient costs (£911 million per year) are dwarfed by the outpatient and community care costs. The total costs to the NHS are of the order of £4.4 billion per year.

There have been considerable advances in our knowledge and understanding of stroke and how to manage it in recent years, particularly with regard to prevention (see Chapters 2, 3 and 11), acute treatment (Chapters 4 and 5) and rehabilitation (Chapters 6–9). Less progress has been achieved in the management of the longer-term issues facing stroke patients and their families (Chapter 12), including psychosocial problems (Chapter 10). These latter topics must form a focus for future service development and research initiatives.

Pathology

About 80–90% of strokes are ischaemic in origin, and 10–20% haemorrhagic. Haemorrhagic strokes tend to be more severe and are associated with higher early mortality. Ischaemic strokes can be classified by the site of the infarct (Table 1.1) or by pathology (Table 1.2). The site of the stroke is of prognostic significance, as illustrated in Figure 1.2. A total anterior circulation infarct has the worst

Table 1.1 Anatomical classification of ischaemic stroke: The Oxford Community Stroke Project.

Lacunar infarcts (LACI)	May cause a 'pure' motor stroke, i.e. a hemi-paresis without loss of sensation or aphasia or visual field defect. May cause a 'pure' sensory stroke, i.e. loss of sensation without motor symptoms. May cause ataxic hemiparesis, i.e. clumsiness. May cause a sensori-motor stroke. Usually associated with small vessel disease.
Total anterior circulation infarcts (TACI)	Causes all of: • new disturbance of higher cerebral dysfunction (e.g dysphasia • hemianopia (partial loss of vision) • severe motor weakness of at least two areas (face, arm or leg) on one side of the body May be associated sensory deficit on one side of the body.
Partial anterior circulation infarcts (PACI)	May cause two of the three components of a TACI. May present with higher cerebral dysfunction alone. May present with a 'pure' motor or sensory deficit that is milder than that associated with a LACI.
Posterior circulation infarcts (POCI)	May cause a cranial nerve palsy and a motor and/or sensory deficit on one side of the body. May cause motor and/or sensory deficit on both sides of the body. May cause visual disturbance (disorder of conjugate eye movement). May cause ataxia (cerebellar dysfunction). May cause isolated partial loss of vision or blindness.

Source: Bamford J, Sandercock P, Dennis M, Burn J, Warlow C. Classification and natural history of clinically identifiable subtypes of cerebral infarction. *Lancet* 1991;**337**:1521–6.

Table 1.2 Pathological classification of ischaemic stroke: The TOAST criteria.

Large artery atherosclerosis	In-situ thrombosis and embolus resulting from atheromatous plaques in the large and medium-sized arteries.
Cardio-embolism	Source of embolus from the heart. Particularly associated with atrial fibrillation. Recent myocardial infarction and prosthetic heart valves important causes.
Small artery disease	Several possible underlying pathologies, of which the commonest is aged-related hyaline arterio-sclerosis of the small vessels supplying the brain.
Other causes	Rarer causes such as haematological and clotting disorders.
Unknown cause	No underlying potential pathology identified.

Source: Adams HP, Bendixen BH, Kappelle LJ, Biller J, Love BB, Gordon DL and Marsh EE. Classification of sub-type of acute ischaemic stroke. Definitions for use in a multi-centre clinical trial. *Stroke* 1993;**24**:35–41.

prognosis, with over 50% mortality at one year and the vast majority of survivors left with significant disability. Over half of ischaemic strokes are caused by embolus, either from the heart or from atheromatous plaques. About a quarter are due to small vessel occlusion (lacunar stroke), and 15% to large vessel athero-thrombosis.

Haemorrhagic strokes most commonly occur in association with hypertension (Box 1.2) and their incidence rises with age due

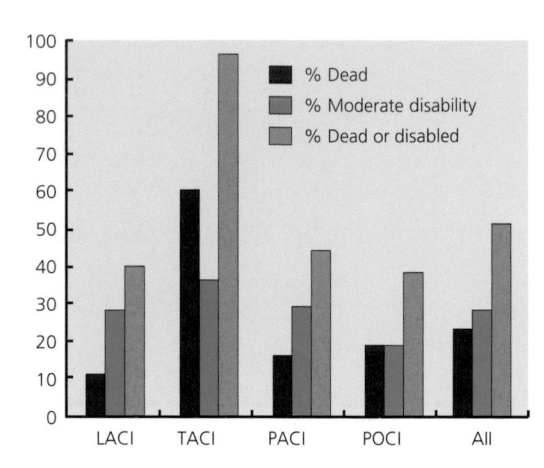

Figure 1.2 Prognosis one year after stroke by site. *Key*: LACI: lacunar infarct; TACI: Total anterior circulation infarct; PACI: Partial anterior circulation infarct; POCI: Posterior circulation infarct. *Source*: Bamford J, Sandercock P, Dennis M, Burn J, Warlow C. Classification and natural history of clinically identifiable subtypes of cerebral infarction. *Lancet* 1991;**337**:1521–56.

to the development of amyloid angiopathy. Another important association of haemorrhagic stroke is antithrombotic treatment with both anticoagulants and antiplatelet agents and thrombolysis (used in the acute treatment of ischaemic stroke and myocardial infarction).

Box 1.2 **Causes of intra-cerebral haemorrhage**

- **Hypertension:** associated with chronic changes in small arteries in brain
- **Amyloid angiopathy:** ageing-associated degenerative changes in small and medium-sized arterial supply to brain characterised by deposition of amyloid ß peptide
- **Antithrombotic therapy:** in particular anticoagulant and antiplatelet therapy
- **Structural abnormalities:** most commonly aneurysms (including sub-arachnoid) and arterio-venous malformations
- **Systemic disease:** clotting factor disorders; blood disorders, including leukaemias
- **Other factors:** alcohol; drugs (amphetamines, cocaine); cerebral tumours

---

Epidemiology

The incidence of first stroke is around 1.5 per 1000 per year, and of transient ischaemic attack 0.6 per 1000 per year. About 22% of all strokes are recurrent events. Stroke incidence rises sharply with age, and is about 1% per annum in people aged 75–84 (Figure 1.3). About 1.5% of the total population have had a past history of stroke or transient ischaemic attack, about 6.7% of people aged 65 or over have had a previous history of stroke and a further 1.3% a history of transient ischaemic attack.

The age-specific incidence of stroke is declining (Figure 1.3), although overall incidence may increase in the future as the proportion of older people in the population rises. Age-standardised mortality from stroke is also declining (Figure 1.4). The decline

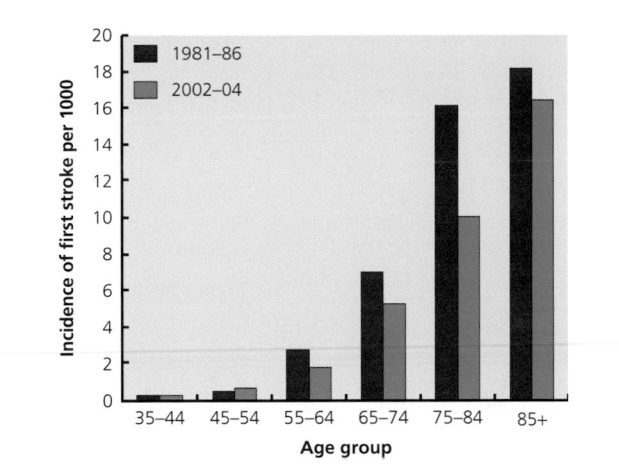

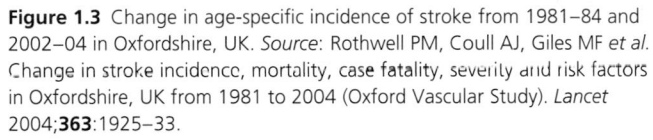

Figure 1.3 Change in age-specific incidence of stroke from 1981–84 and 2002–04 in Oxfordshire, UK. *Source*: Rothwell PM, Coull AJ, Giles MF *et al.* Change in stroke incidence, mortality, case fatality, severity and risk factors in Oxfordshire, UK from 1981 to 2004 (Oxford Vascular Study). *Lancet* 2004;**363**:1925–33.

in stroke mortality has been steeper than the decline in all-cause mortality. This reflects both the fall in incidence and improvement in survival following stroke. The downward trend goes back to the early part of the twentieth century, and is likely to reflect a combination of improvements in population health through better living conditions, changes in diet (e.g. less use of salt as a preservative; greater use of polyunsaturated fats) and, more recently, introduction of medical interventions such as antihypertensives and statins.

Risk factors for stroke

Several factors have been identified that are associated with an increased risk of stroke; see Table 1.3. The importance of a risk factor is determined both by its frequency in the population and the strength of its association with stroke (as measured by the size of the relative risk). In these terms, *hypertension, smoking* and *atrial fibrillation* can be regarded as the most important risk factors for stroke – the first two because of their high prevalence and the latter both because of its high prevalence in the elderly (see Chapter 2) and its very strong association with stroke (Table 1.3).

There is considerable overlap between the risk factors for stroke and the risk factors for ischaemic heart disease. There are differences as well, however. The two most striking of these are:

- the stronger association between blood pressure and stroke risk than blood pressure and ischaemic heart disease;
- the apparent non-association between serum cholesterol level and risk of stroke in contrast to its strong association with risk of ischaemic heart disease.

The differences largely reflect the fact that 'stroke' is an umbrella term with a heterogeneous mix of underlying pathologies, only some of which (i.e. large artery atherosclerosis and cardio-embolism) are related to the pathology of ischaemic heart disease.

Sociodemographic

Although for a given age men are at a higher risk of stroke than women, overall women account for more strokes than men because of their longer life expectancy and the close association of stroke risk with age. The association of socio-economic status with stroke risk is due to a combination of individual lifestyle factors (e.g. smoking and alcohol consumption) and adverse living circumstances (e.g. poorer housing).

Biological

The key biological risk factor for stroke is blood pressure. Long-term epidemiological studies have challenged the concept of 'hypertension' as a discrete condition, demonstrating that lower

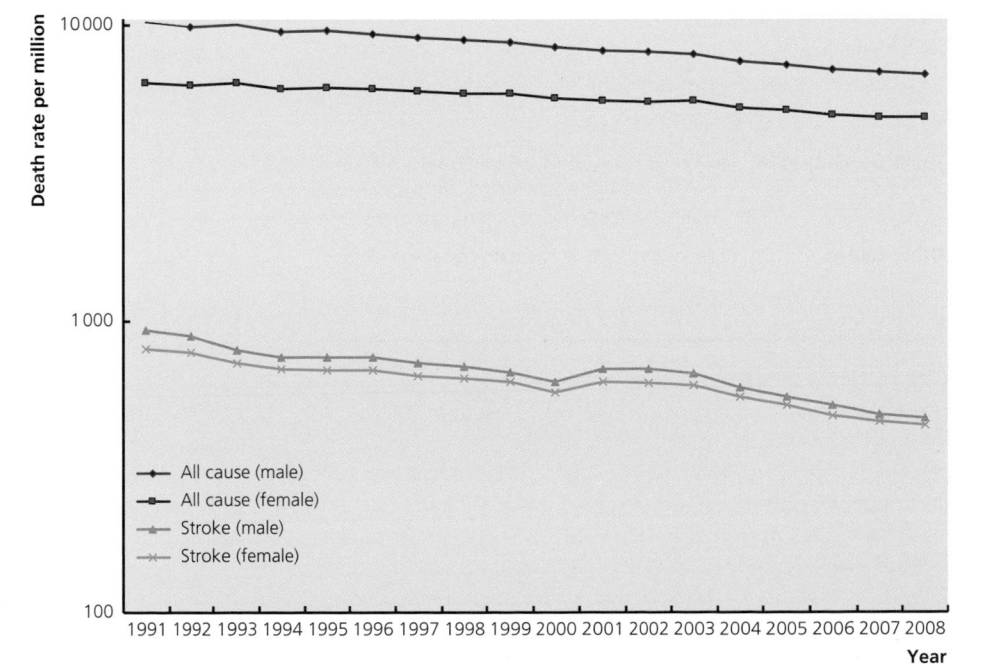

Figure 1.4 Mortality trends for all cause and stroke in England and Wales, 1991–2008. *Note*: Death rates are directly standardised to the European Standard population. *Data source*: Office for National Statistics. Mortality statistics: Deaths registered in 2008. Review of the National Statistician on deaths in England & Wales 2008. Series DR, Crown Copyright 2009.

Table 1.3 Risk factors for stroke.

Sociodemographic	• Age (see Figure 1.5) • Sex (see Figures 1.4 and 1.5): slightly higher risk in men • Ethnicity: higher risk in African Caribbean and South Asian populations • Socio-economic status: increasing deprivation is associated with increased risk
Biological	• Raised blood pressure: doubling in risk of death from stroke for every 10 mmHg increase in diastolic blood pressure or 20 mmHg increase in systolic blood pressure • Hypercholesterolaemia • Hyperhomocysteinaemia
Lifestyle	• Smoking: 50% increase in risk • Excessive alcohol consumption: 50–100% increase in risk • Physical inactivity: 2.5-fold increase in risk • Diet: obesity; low potassium; high salt; low fruit and vegetable intake
Other conditions	• Diabetes mellitus: doubling of risk • Atrial fibrillation: fivefold increase in risk • Ischaemic heart disease: doubling in risk • Cardiac sources of thrombo-embolism • Haematological disorders: sickle cell disease; raised packed cell volume; hypercoagulability • Carotid artery stenosis • Migraine
Genetic	• Positive family history in parents: 50–100% increase in risk • 2 single nucleotide polymorphisms (SNPs) on choromosome 12p13 associated with 40% increase in risk
Other factors	• Oral contraception: doubling of risk • Hormone replacement therapy: doubling of risk • Major life events • Influenza and other intercurrent infections

blood pressures (at least down to a systolic blood pressure of 115 mmHg) are associated with a lower risk of stroke (and ischaemic heart disease). Randomised controlled trials have demonstrated that in people at high risk of vascular events, even those with 'normal' blood pressure benefit from having their blood pressure lowered.

Although epidemiological studies have not demonstrated significant associations between cholesterol and stroke risk, the strong evidence from randomised controlled trials that cholesterol lowering with statins lowers stroke risk suggests that there is a causal association.

Conversely, although epidemiological studies have shown a link between raised serum homocysteine levels and risk of stroke, randomised controlled trials have not unequivocally demonstrated that lowering homocysteine (through folate supplementation) leads to reduced stroke risk.

Lifestyle

The lifestyle factors are partly mediated through their effect on blood pressure (e.g. salt, exercise, obesity) and cholesterol (e.g. exercise and obesity), but also partly through other independent effects

on atheroma development. The association between alcohol and stroke is complex, in that low levels of alcohol consumption are associated with a lower risk of stroke than complete abstinence. The extent to which this demonstrates a genuine protective effect of alcohol or reflects confounding by other factors (e.g. conditions that might be associated with non-drinking) is unclear.

Other conditions and factors

Not surprisingly, existing cardiovascular disease and diabetes are strong risk factors for stroke.

It can be difficult to disentangle the extent to which family history as a risk factor reflects shared exposure to environmental risk factors or genetic predisposition. Recent genome-wide association studies have, however, found strong associations with a couple of gene loci, suggesting that genetic factors do play a part.

Given that the absolute risks of stroke are low in women of an age likely to be taking the oral contraceptive pill, or indeed hormone replacement therapy (see Figure 1.5), the increased risk of stroke associated with these agents only comes into play if there are other risk factors, such as migraine and hypertension.

Observational studies have demonstrated links between upper respiratory tract infections and risk of stroke, and between influenza vaccination and decreased risk of stroke. The explanation for this link remains unclear, though it is plausible that such infections might result in short-term increases in risk.

Prognosis

Overall survival rates following stroke are of the order of 20–30% after one month and 30–40% after one year. However, such aggregated rates are of little meaning for an individual, given that survival is dependent on a host of factors, such as:

- Type of stroke (Figure 1.2)
- Age
- Stroke severity – can be measured in a number of ways. Simple features such as incontinence and inability to swallow are associated with poorer survival

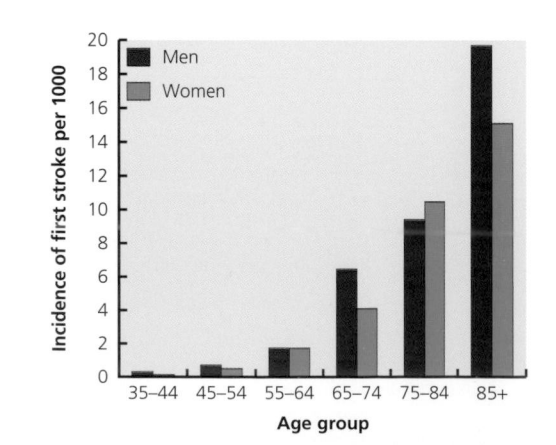

Figure 1.5 Incidence of stroke by age and sex. *Source*: Rothwell PM, Coull AJ, Giles MF *et al*. Change in stroke incidence, mortality, case fatality, severity and risk factors in Oxfordshire, UK from 1981 to 2004 (Oxford Vascular Study). *Lancet* 2004;**363**:1925–33.

- Ethnicity – better prognosis in the African Caribbean population compared to the white population
- Atrial fibrillation – associated with more severe strokes
- Co-morbidity – such as prior stroke or diabetes, associated with worse survival.

Physical recovery as measured by ability to perform the activities of daily living is usually maximal by six months after stroke, although more complex aspects of physical recovery such as speech and language abilities may improve over years. Good epidemiological studies of such aspects of stroke recovery are sparse. Advances in brain imaging such as functional Magnetic Resonance Imaging (fMRI) have provided insights into how the brain can relearn functions initially lost after a stroke, and have provided grounds for greater therapeutic optimism than was the case in the past, when it was perhaps assumed that the adult brain had limited 'plasticity'; that is, it was unable to use different parts to take over functions lost following stroke.

Further reading

Donnan GA, Fisher M, Macleod M, Davis SM. Stroke. *Lancet* 2008;**371**: 1612–23.

Mant J, Wade DT, Winner S. Health care needs assessment: Stroke. In: (eds) Stevens A, Raftery J, Mant J, Simpson S. *Health Care Needs Assessment: The Epidemiologically Based Needs Assessment Reviews*, First series, 2nd edn, pp 141–244. Oxford: Radcliffe Medical Press, 2004. http://www.hcna.bham.ac.uk/chapters.shtml.

Qureshi AI, Mendelow AD, Hanley DF. Intra-cerebral haemorrhage. *Lancet* 2009;**373**:1632–44.

CHAPTER 2

Primary Prevention of Stroke

Jonathan Mant

Addenbrooke's Hospital, University of Cambridge, UK

OVERVIEW

- Population-based approaches and identification and treatment of 'high-risk' individuals are complementary strategies for stroke prevention
- Cardiovascular risk can be calculated for an individual using a combination of several individual risk factors, including blood pressure and serum cholesterol
- Smoking, diet, exercise and alcohol consumption are important modifiable aspects of lifestyle
- Drug treatment to reduce risk of stroke focuses on cholesterol and blood pressure lowering
- The risk of stroke associated with atrial fibrillation can be substantially reduced through anticoagulation

There is considerable overlap between prevention of stroke and prevention of coronary heart disease. Two activities specific to stroke prevention are the use of antithrombotic therapy for atrial fibrillation and surgery for carotid artery stenosis.

There are two complementary approaches to stroke prevention: population-based approaches, where the aim is to lower the level of a risk factor in the whole population; and individual-based approaches, where the aim is to identify and treat risk factors in people at high risk of disease. Neither approach should be ignored.

Population approaches

Population-based strategies have the potential for much greater impact than the identification and treatment of 'high-risk' individuals, simply because the majority of cardiovascular events occur in people who are not identified as being at high risk. Another attraction of the population-based approach is that it tends to reduce the number of 'high-risk' individuals – for example, if the mean alcohol consumption of the whole population is reduced, there are likely to be fewer people who exceed safe drinking thresholds.

Population approaches include strategies to make environmental and socio-economic conditions more favourable to health and strategies to influence behaviour in such a way that 'healthy' choices

are more likely to be made. Examples of population approaches include:

- Legislation: banning tobacco advertising; provision of smoke-free environments
- Taxation: raising price of 'unhealthy' lifestyles such as smoking and drinking
- Advertising campaigns: awareness raising
- Environmental: provision of environments to exercise safely (e.g. safe cycling and walking routes)
- Information: clearer food labelling
- Reduction of salt in processed foods

There is a political dimension to some of these population strategies – raising taxes is rarely popular and concerns have been raised over 'social engineering'. There is a deeper philosophical question about the extent to which health is determined by individual choice or by broader socio-economic and environmental factors that are better influenced by government.

Use of pharmacological treatments such as statins and antihypertensives have traditionally been viewed as appropriate only for 'high-risk' individuals, but this orthodoxy is being challenged by the concept of a 'polypill', whereby all people over a certain age (age being a very simple and strong risk factor for stroke) might be offered medication purely because of their age rather than because of the presence of any risk factors. The potential role of this approach is being explored in a number of studies worldwide.

Identification of people at high risk of stroke

There are many potential risk factors for stroke (see Chapter 1). Several of these factors have been combined into risk scores based on analysis of cohort studies. These scores enable the future risk of a cardiovascular event to be calculated (see Table 2.1). Currently, a cut-off of greater than 20% risk over 10 years is used to identify those who should be offered drug therapy. The Framingham risk score has been in use for over 20 years, but has limitations in that it does not take into account factors such as social deprivation, family history and ethnicity. The QRISK2 score was developed on a larger dataset than the other scores, so was able to identify independent roles of factors such as obesity (as measured by Body Mass Index),

---

ABC of Stroke. Edited by Jonathan Mant and Marion F Walker.
© 2011 Blackwell Publishing Ltd.

Table 2.1 Components of three cardiovascular risk scores commonly used in the UK.

Risk factor	Framingham 1991 http://www.framinghamheartstudy.org/risk/index.html*	ASSIGN http://assign-score.com/	QRISK2 http://www.qrisk.org/
Socio-demographic			
Age	YES	YES	YES
Sex	YES	YES	YES
Ethnicity	NO	NO	YES self assigned – white; Indian; Pakistani; Bangladeshi; other Asian; black African; black Caribbean; Chinese; Other (inc. mixed)
Social deprivation	NO	YES Scottish Index of multiple deprivation (uses postcode)	YES Townsend deprivation score (uses postcode)
Biological			
Blood pressure	YES systolic	YES systolic	YES systolic
Blood lipid levels	YES ratio TC:HDL	YES TC & HDL separately	YES ratio TC:HDL
Body Mass Index	NO	NO	YES
Left Ventricular Hypertrophy	YES +ve if ECG criteria met	NO	NO
Lifestyle			
Smoking status	YES +ve if current smoker or stopped within last year	YES number of cigarettes smoked daily	YES current or non-smoker, including ex-smoker
Existing diagnoses			
Treated hypertension	NO	NO	YES +ve if diagnosis of hypertension and at least one prescription for an antihypertensive
Rheumatoid arthritis	NO	NO	YES
Chronic renal disease	NO	NO	YES
Diabetes mellitus	YES diabetes	YES diabetes	YES type 2 diabetes
Atrial fibrillation	NO	NO	YES
Genetic			
Family history	NO	YES +ve if coronary heart disease or stroke in close relative under 60 years	YES +ve if coronary heart disease in first-degree relative under 60 years

Key: YES/NO indicates whether or not risk factor is included; ratio TC:HDL – ratio of total serum cholesterol/high-density lipoprotein cholesterol

Note: *This web link is to a more recent Framingham score than the 1991 score, but it is the 1991 score that is more widely used in the UK.

Adapted from:
Anderson KM, Odell PM, Wilson PW, Kannel WB. Cardiovascular disease risk profiles. *Am Heart J* 1991;**121**:293–8.
Woodward M, Brindle P, Tunstall-Pedoe, H. Adding social deprivation and family history to cardiovascular risk assessment: The ASSIGN score from the Scottish Heart Health Extended Cohort (SHHEC). *Heart* 2007;**93**:172–6.
Hippisley-Cox J, Coupland C, Vinogradova Y, Robson J, Brindle P. Predicting cardiovascular risk in England and Wales: Prospective derivation and validation of QRISK2. *BMJ* 2008;**336**:1475–82.

atrial fibrillation and rheumatoid arthritis. The core risk factors for cardiovascular disease – blood pressure; cholesterol; smoking and diabetes – are common to all the scores.

Lifestyle modification

Aspects of lifestyle that are associated with a lower risk of cardiovascular disease are well known and widely accepted (see Figure 2.1 and Table 2.2). Differences in lifestyle are associated with substantial differences in cardiovascular risk. For example:

- Someone eating five or more portions of fruit and vegetable per day has a 26% lower risk of stroke than someone who eats fewer than three
- A smoker has a 1.5 times higher risk of having a stroke than a non-smoker
- Reducing salt consumption from 10 g to 5 g a day (equivalent of a teaspoon of salt) will reduce blood pressure by about 5 mmHg.
- A physically inactive person is at over double the risk of a stroke than a physically active person

Drug treatment

Blood pressure lowering

People with a sustained blood pressure of over 160/100 mmHg or with a blood pressure of over 140/90 mmHg with a 10-year risk of developing cardiovascular disease of over 20% should be started on drug therapy to lower blood pressure (see Figure 2.2). Lowering blood pressure leads to important reductions in the risk of both stroke and heart disease. In the randomised trials of blood pressure-lowering therapy, lowering systolic blood pressure by 10 mmHg (or diastolic blood pressure by 5 mmHg) was associated with a 41% reduction in stroke risk and a 22% reduction in coronary heart disease risk.

Cholesterol lowering

People with raised cardiovascular risk should be offered treatment with a statin. There is some controversy over whether this should be at a fixed dose, or titrated to a treatment target based on total cholesterol and low-density lipoprotein cholesterol (LDL cholesterol) – see Box 2.1. Nevertheless, the findings of the Heart

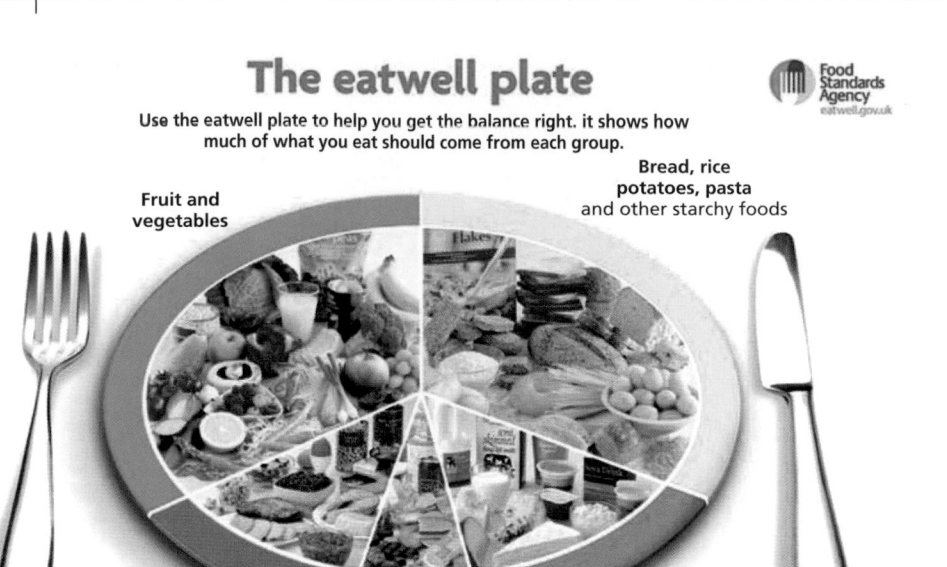

Figure 2.1 A healthy well-balanced diet. Reproduced under the terms of the Click-Use Licence. *Source*: Food Standards Agency, Crown copyright 2010.

Table 2.2 Lifestyle modification to lower cardiovascular risk.

Diet	• Restrict total fat intake (to 30% or less of total energy intake) • Replace saturated fats with monosaturated and polyunsaturated fats • Eat at least five portions of fruit and vegetables per day • Eat at least two portions of fish per week, including an oily fish (salmon, trout, herring, pilchards, sardines, fresh tuna) • Reduce salt intake • Weight loss if overweight or obese
Physical activity	• Moderate physical activity (sufficient to become slightly breathless) for 20–30 minutes daily
Alcohol consumption	• Keep within recognised safe drinking limits: 3–4 units per day for men; 2–3 units per day for women • Avoid binge drinking
Smoking cessation	• Can be facilitated by pharmacological agents and psychological support

Sources: The National Collaborating Centre for Primary Care. Lipid Modification: Cardiovascular risk assessment and the modification of blood lipids for the primary and secondary prevention of cardiovascular disease. Full Guideline. Royal College of General Practitioners, London. May 2008. Intercollegiate Stroke Working Party. *National Clinical Guideline for Stroke*, 3rd edn. London: Royal College of Physicians, 2008.

Protection Study suggest that taking 40 mg of simvastatin a day will lead to a 1.5 mmol/l reduction in LDL cholesterol, which would reduce the risk of cardiovascular events by about a third. The results of a meta-analysis of randomised controlled trials of statins underline the significant benefits of treatment with this class of drug (Table 2.3). Long-term follow-up of one of these trials, the West of Scotland Coronary Prevention Study, found that the benefits of statin therapy were sustained for 10 years after the trial ended, even though after the trial finished similar proportions of the intervention and control groups were being treated with statins.

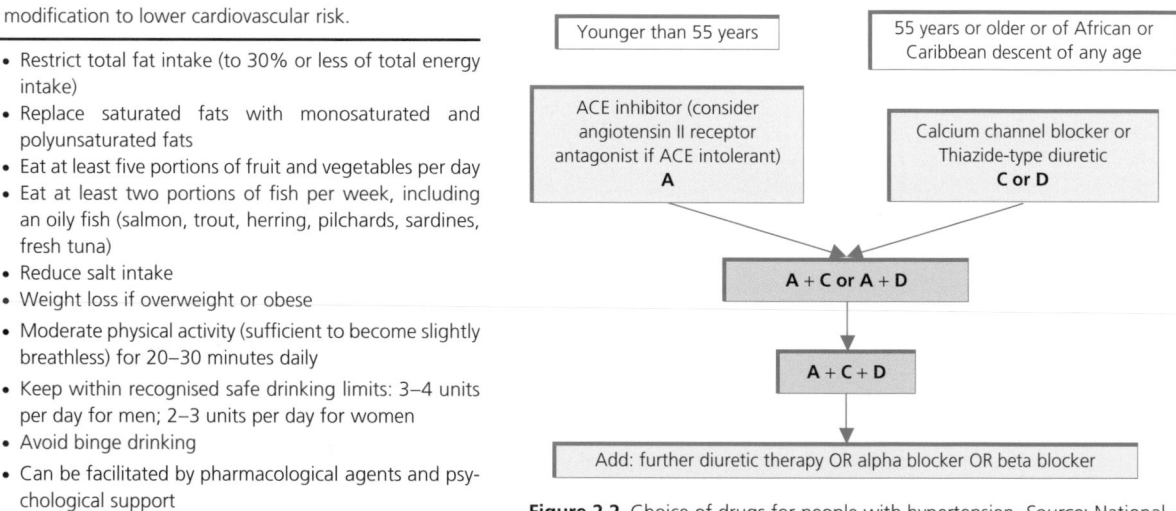

Figure 2.2 Choice of drugs for people with hypertension. *Source*: National Institute for Health and Clinical Excellence. *Hypertension: Management of hypertension in adults in primary care.* NICE Clinical Guideline no 34, London 2006.

This suggests that statins do slow (or possibly even reverse) the development of atherosclerosis.

> **Box 2.1 Conflicting guidance on cholesterol lowering for primary prevention of cardiovascular disease: Treat to target or 'fire and forget'?**
>
> **NICE recommends** a 'fire and forget' strategy for primary prevention of cardiovascular disease in adults who have a 20% or greater 10-year risk of a cardiovascular event. This entails commencing simvastatin 40 mg, and not subsequently monitoring serum lipid levels or increasing the dose or using a higher-intensity statin.

The Joint British Societies recommend a 'treat to target' strategy for adults with a 20% or greater 10-year risk of a cardiovascular event, titrating lipid-modifying drugs to achieve a total cholesterol target of less than 4.0 mmol/l and low-density lipoprotein cholesterol (LDL) target of less than 2.0 mmol/l, with serum lipid levels monitored at least annually.

The controversy revolves around the extent to which it is appropriate or not to extrapolate from randomised controlled trials in secondary prevention or to rely on indirect evidence from epidemiological analyses.

- Is intensification of lipid-lowering therapy effective? The evidence that higher doses of lipid-modifying therapy lead to better outcome is in people with existing coronary heart disease. There is no direct evidence for intensification of lipid-lowering therapy in primary prevention. However, there is circumstantial evidence: the trials that achieved larger reductions in LDL cholesterol were associated with bigger reductions in risk of cardiovascular events, and observational studies show that lower total cholesterol and LDL cholesterol levels are associated with lower risk of subsequent cardiovascular events.

- Is it appropriate to set a target level for cholesterol? Again, there have been no trials of different target levels in primary prevention. A justification for targets can be made on the observational epidemiological evidence that lower total cholesterol (down to at least 4 mmol/L) is associated with lower risk of cardiovascular events.

- Is there value in monitoring serum lipid levels after drug treatment has been initiated? This is necessary if a 'treat to target' strategy is being employed, and is also of possible benefit as a means of monitoring and improving adherence to therapy.

- Which strategy offers better value for money? Modelling work done for NICE suggested that for secondary prevention, 'treat to target' was cost effective in that the additional cost of treatment and monitoring was justified in terms of the better outcomes that were achieved. It is not clear which strategy would provide best value for money for primary prevention.

Adapted from: The National Collaborating Centre for Primary Care. Lipid Modification: Cardiovascular risk assessment and the modification of blood lipids for the primary and secondary prevention of cardiovascular disease. Full Guideline. Royal College of General Practitioners, London. May 2008.

JBS 2: Joint British Societies' guidelines on prevention of cardiovascular disease in clinical practice Prepared by: British Cardiac Society, British Hypertension Society, Diabetes UK, HEART UK, Primary Care Cardiovascular Society, The Stroke Association. *Heart* 2005;**91**:v1–v52. doi: 10.1136/hrt.2005.079988.

Antiplatelet therapy

The pendulum has recently swung away from the use of antiplatelet agents for the primary prevention of stroke. Given the emergence of statins as an effective agent for primary prevention and improvements in blood pressure control in recent years, the additional benefit of aspirin has declined in absolute terms, such that it is not clear that the benefit of prevention of cardiovascular events is not neutralised by the increased risk of bleeding (see Box 2.2). Ongoing trials will clarify whether aspirin is still indicated for primary prevention in specific high-risk groups such as people with diabetes.

Table 2.3 Effects of 1 mmol/l reduction in LDL cholesterol by statins: Results from a meta-analysis of data from 90 056 participants in 14 randomised trials of statins.

	Treatment	Control	RR (CI)
Deaths			
Any	8.5%	9.7%	0.88 (0.84–0.91)
Vascular	4.7%	5.7%	0.83 (0.79–0.87)
Non-vascular	3.8%	4.0%	0.95 (0.90–1.01)
Strokes			
Any	3.0%	3.7%	0.83 (0.78–0.88)
Ischaemic	2.8%	3.4%	0.81 (0.74–0.89)
Haemorrhagic	0.2%	0.2%	1.05 (0.78–1.41)
Major coronary events			
Non-fatal MI	4.4%	6.2%	0.74 (0.70–0.79)
CHD death	3.4%	4.4%	0.81 (0.75–0.87)

Note: Mean duration of follow-up: 4.7 years.
Key: RR (CI): Relative risk and 95% confidence interval
Source: Cholesterol Treatment Trialists' (CTT) Collaborators. Efficacy and safety of cholesterol-lowering treatment: Prospective meta-analysis of data from 90 056 participants in 14 randomised trials of statins. *Lancet* 2005;**366**: 1267–78.

Box 2.2 **Aspirin for primary prevention?**

Aspirin reduces the risk of serious vascular events, with a relative risk of a vascular event of 0.88 for someone on aspirin as compared to a placebo. In randomised controlled trials of primary prevention, this equates to annual risks of 0.51% versus 0.57% – a 0.06% reduction in risk in absolute terms; that is, a number needed to treat (NNT) of 1667 for one year to prevent one event. The benefit is mostly in terms of reduction of non-fatal myocardial infarction. There is no effect on stroke risk if haemorrhagic strokes are taken into account.

The potential for harm needs to be set against this small reduction in the risk of vascular events. Aspirin increases the risk of major gastrointestinal and extra-cranial bleeds, with a relative risk of 1.54 for someone on aspirin as compared to a placebo. The rates of major haemorrhage in the trials are 0.10% versus 0.07% per annum – a 0.03% increase in risk in absolute terms.

Thus, on the face of it, aspirin would appear to prevent two major vascular events per major haemorrhage caused. However, risks of stroke and other vascular events have declined since these trials were performed (see Chapter 1), in part because of the emergence of statins. Conversely, it is unlikely that there has been any secular change in the risk of haemorrhage. If the risk of a cardiovascular event has halved because of the use of other drugs, then the ratio of harm to benefit reduces to about one to one, which is not a clear justification for aspirin therapy for primary prevention.

While it might be tempting to consider using a cardiovascular risk threshold to determine which people might be offered aspirin therapy, in practice a major determinant of risk of a cardiovascular event is age, which is also a major determinant of risk of haemorrhage. Thus, older people potentially have more to gain from aspirin therapy, but also have more to lose.

Source: Antithrombotic Trialists' Collaboration. Aspirin in the primary and secondary prevention of vascular disease: Collaborative meta-analysis of individual participant data from randomised trials. *Lancet* 2009;**373**:1849–60.

Management of stroke-specific risk factors

Atrial fibrillation

Atrial fibrillation, characterised clinically by an 'irregularly irregular' pulse, is an important cause of stroke, particularly in older people, with a prevalence of around 7% in people aged 65 or over and 12% in those aged 75 or over. It is becoming more common as a result of improved survival of people with ischaemic heart disease, which is its major cause. It may be asymptomatic, and thus active screening can detect new cases. Opportunistic screening by pulse palpation followed by ECG if the pulse is irregular is the recommended approach, as it detects as many cases as systematic screening by ECG (see Figure 2.3).

There are two main treatment options to reduce stroke risk in atrial fibrillation: use of antiplatelet agents such as aspirin and use of anticoagulants such as warfarin, which requires regular blood tests to monitor treatment (INR – International Normalised Ratio – tests). Guidelines recommend that the decision of which to use is informed by an assessment of the individual's risk of stroke. The tool most widely used is the CHADS2 score (Table 2.4), which assigns people a score between 0 and 6 on the basis of simple clinical features. The scores are often grouped into three categories, with anticoagulation the preferred treatment for high risk, antiplatelet therapy for low risk, and either treatment for people at moderate risk. In practice, clinical decision making is a little more complex, as risk of bleeding (the major side effect of warfarin) needs to be taken into account.

One of the major risk factors for bleeding is increase in age. Concern about this has limited the use of anticoagulation in the elderly, but recent evidence from the Birmingham Atrial Fibrillation

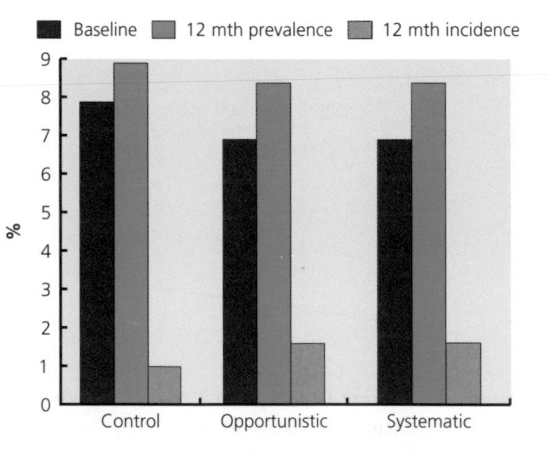

Figure 2.3 Prevalence and detection rates of new cases of atrial fibrillation (AF) in people aged >65.

Note: Figure shows baseline (i.e. before any screening carried out) prevalence of AF, prevalence after one year of screening and incidence (new cases of AF detected over that one-year period). Three different strategies were tested:

- Control: no active screening was carried out.
- Opportunistic: practice staff were encouraged to take the pulse of people aged over 64 when they attended the practice for any reason. If the pulse was found to be irregular, then the patient would be offered an ECG.
- Systematic: people aged over 64 were invited to attend the practice for an ECG.

Source: Fitzmaurice DA, Hobbs FDR, Jowett S *et al*. Screening versus routine practice in detection of atrial fibrillation in patients aged 65 or over: Cluster randomised controlled trial. *BMJ* 2007;**335**:383. doi:10.1136/bmj.39280.660567.55.

Table 2.4 The CHADS2 score.

Components	Score
Recent **C**ongestive heart failure	1 pt
Hypertension	1 pt
Age 75 or over	1 pt
Diabetes mellitus	1 pt
Prior **S**troke or transient ischaemic attack	2 pts
TOTAL	Score between 0 and 6

Interpretation	
High risk	2 or more points
Moderate risk	1 point
Low risk	0 points

Source: Gage BF, Waterman AD, Shannon W, Boechler M, Rich MW, Radford MJ. Validation of clinical classification schemes for predicting stroke: Results from the national registry of atrial fibrillation. *JAMA* 2001;**285**:2864–70.

Treatment of the Aged trial (BAFTA) has demonstrated that warfarin is superior to aspirin in this age group (see Box 2.3).

Box 2.3 **Summary of the BAFTA trial**

The table shows the risks per annum of events (primary event, major extra-cranial haemorrhage and death) in people randomised to warfarin or aspirin.

- **Study population:** 973 people aged 75 or over (mean age 81) with atrial fibrillation recruited from general practices in England and Wales; mean follow-up 2.7 years
- **Interventions:** warfarin (target INR 2–3) or aspirin (75 mg daily)
- **Primary end-point:** fatal or disabling stroke (ischaemic or haemorrhagic), intracranial haemorrhage or clinically significant arterial embolism
- **Secondary outcome:** major extra-cranial haemorrhage: fatal, or one that resulted in the need for transfusion or surgery
- **Key results:**

	Warfarin	Aspirin	RR, 95% CI	P value	NNT
Primary end-point	1.8%	3.8%	0.48, 0.28–0.80	0.0027	50
Major haemorrhage	1.4%	1.6%	0.87, 0.43–1.73	0.67	–
Death	8.0%	8.4%	0.95, 0.72–1.26	0.73	–

Key: RR: relative risk; 95% CI: 95% confidence interval; NNT: number needed to treat to prevent one event if treated with warfarin rather than aspirin for one year

Source: Mant J, Hobbs FD, Fletcher K *et al*. Warfarin versus aspirin for stroke prevention in atrial fibrillation in the elderly community population: The Birmingham Atrial Fibrillation Treatment of the Aged Study (BAFTA), a randomised controlled trial. *Lancet* 2007;**370**:493–503.

Newer anticoagulants that do not require regular blood tests are being developed to mitigate the inconvenience of warfarin therapy. The most promising of these to date is dabigatran, which was evaluated in the RE-LY trial (see Box 2.4).

Carotid artery stenosis

Carotid artery stenosis – that is, narrowing of the carotid artery caused by atherosclerosis – increases the risk of stroke. This risk

Box 2.4 **Summary of the RE-LY trial**

The table shows the risks per annum of events (primary event, major extra-cranial haemorrhage and death) in people randomised to dabigatran or warfarin.

- **Study population:** 18 113 people (mean age 71) with atrial fibrillation and another risk factor for stroke; mean follow-up 2.0 years
- **Interventions:** warfarin (target INR 2–3) or dabigatran 110 mg or 150 mg twice daily
- **Primary end-point:** stroke or systemic embolism
- **Secondary outcome:** major haemorrhage: significant fall in haemoglobin ($\geq$20 g/l), transfusion of at least 2 units of blood, or symptomatic bleeding in critical area or organ
- **Key results:**

	Dabigatran		Warfarin	RR, 95% CI		NNT	
	D1 110 mg	D2 150 mg		D1 v W	D2 v W	D1 v W	D2 v W
Primary end-point	1.5%	1.1%	1.7%	0.91, 0.74–1.11	0.66, 0.53–0.82	–	167
Major haemorrhage	2.7%	3.1%	3.4%	0.80, 0.69–0.93	0.93, 0.81–1.07	334	–
Death	3.7%	3.6%	4.1%	0.91, 0.80–1.03	0.88, 0.77–1.00	–	–

Key: RR: relative risk; 95% CI: 95% confidence interval; NNT: number needed to treat to prevent one event if treated with dabigatran rather than warfarin for one year
Source: Connolly SJ, Ezekowitz MD, Yusufet S *et al*. Dabigatran versus warfarin in patients with atrial fibrillation. *N Engl J Med* 2009;**361**:1139–51.

Table 2.5 Cochrane Review of Trials of Carotid Endarterectomy for asymptomatic carotid stenosis.

Description of studies	Three trials involving 5223 patients followed up for an average of 3.3 years Publication dates: 1993, 1995, 2004 Mean age: 67 years All involved randomisation to carotid endarterectomy (including antiplatelet therapy) or standard medical care (including antiplatelet therapy)
Outcomes	
1 Perioperative stroke or death	2.9%
2 Perioperative stroke or death or subsequent stroke (primary outcome)	31% relative risk reduction with surgery (RR: 0.69, 95% CI 0.57–0.83), p < 0.0001
3 Absolute risk reduction of primary outcome	1.0% over 4 years (1993 publication) 3.0% over 2.7 years (1995 publication) 3.1% over 3.4 years (2004 publication)
4 Number of operations needed to prevent one stroke	100 to prevent 1 stroke in 4 years (1993) 33 to prevent 1 stroke in 2.7 years (1995) 32 to prevent 1 stroke in 3.4 years (2004)

Key: RR: relative risk; 95% CI: 95% confidence interval
Source: Chambers BR, Donnan G. Carotid endarterectomy for asymptomatic carotid stenosis. *Cochrane Database of Systematic Reviews* 2005, Issue 4. CD001923, DOI: 10.1002/14651858.CD001923.pub2.

can be reduced by carotid endarterectomy, surgical removal of the stenosed part of the carotid artery. This operation has a clear role in people who have had a previous stroke or transient ischaemic attack (see Chapters 3 and 11), but its place in the management of people found to have carotid artery stenosis who have not had a stroke or transient ischaemic attack is less clear cut. There is a perioperative risk of stroke or death of the order of 3%, and while randomised controlled trials have demonstrated that the long-term benefit of surgery more than outweighs this short-term harm, the

absolute benefit from treatment observed in the trials was small (see Table 2.5). For example, in the Medical Research Council Trial published in 2004, 32 operations would be required to prevent one stroke over a 3.4-year follow-up period. Furthermore, this benefit is likely to be still lower in people treated with current optimal medical therapy (antiplatelet agents, statins and antihypertensives). There have been no trials of population screening for carotid endarterectomy.

A less invasive treatment of carotid artery stenosis, carotid artery stenting (insertion of a tube under x-ray control to open up the narrowed artery) has been developed. However, results from randomised controlled trials suggest that this will only have a limited role to play, in that it is associated with a higher risk of perioperative stroke than endarterectomy (though lower risk of perioperative myocardial infarction).

Further reading

Ford I, Murray H, Packard CJ, Shepherd J, Macfarlane PW, Cobbe SM for the West of Scotland Coronary Prevention Study Group. Long-Term Follow-up of the West of Scotland Coronary Prevention Study. *N Engl J Med* 2007;**357**:1477–86.

Heart Protection Study Collaborative Group. MRC/BHF Heart Protection Study of cholesterol lowering with simvastatin in 20 536 high-risk individuals: A randomised placebo controlled trial. *Lancet* 2002;**360**:7–22.

Mant J, Edwards D. Stroke prevention in atrial fibrillation: Putting the guidelines into practice. *Drugs & Aging* 2010;**27**(11):859–70.

The National Collaborating Centre for Primary Care. Lipid Modification: Cardiovascular risk assessment and the modification of blood lipids for the primary and secondary prevention of cardiovascular disease. Full Guideline. Royal College of General Practitioners, London. May 2008.

Wald NJ, Law MR. A strategy to reduce cardiovascular disease by more than 80%. *BMJ* 2003;**326**:1419–25.

CHAPTER 3

Transient Ischaemic Attack

Jonathan Mant

Addenbrooke's Hospital, University of Cambridge, UK

OVERVIEW

- About 1 person per 1000 per year will suffer a transient ischaemic attack (TIA) or minor stroke that is treated as a TIA
- The risk of a stroke after a TIA is high, particularly in the first few days
- A simple clinical score (ABCD^2) can predict which patients are at very high risk of stroke following a TIA
- Prompt medical therapy of a TIA may have a substantial effect in reducing the risk of stroke
- Urgent carotid endarterectomy is necessary if the TIA is associated with significant carotid artery stenosis

A transient ischaemic attack (TIA) is traditionally defined as an acute loss of focal cerebral or ocular function with symptoms lasting less than 24 hours, which is caused by embolic or thrombotic vascular disease. The distinction between TIA and stroke is one of duration of symptoms, with 24 hours representing a watershed between the two. This distinction is arbitrary – some patients with symptoms lasting less than 24 hours have evidence of infarction on brain imaging, and others with more protracted symptoms have no such evidence. Clinically, the distinction does not matter since the management of TIA and minor stroke is essentially the same. The incidence of TIA and minor stroke that presents like a TIA is of the order of 1 per 1000 people per year.

Prognosis following TIA

About a quarter of patients with ischaemic stroke have a TIA first, and over 40% of these occur in the week preceding the stroke. In the past, the risks of stroke following TIA were under-estimated, since studies tended not to capture the TIAs that occurred in close temporal proximity to a stroke, and therefore reported a falsely benign prognosis. The true risk of stroke following an untreated TIA is around 8% after 7 days and 17% after 90 days, with the risks following a minor stroke a little higher (Figure 3.1).

The individual risk following a TIA varies considerably, depending on simple clinical features (how long the TIA lasts, and whether or not it leads to unilateral weakness or speech disturbance) and

ABC of Stroke. Edited by Jonathan Mant and Marion F Walker.
© 2011 Blackwell Publishing Ltd.

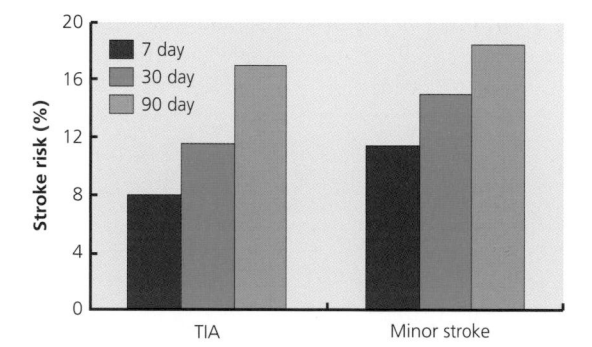

Figure 3.1 Risk of stroke following TIA and minor stroke. *Source*: Data from Coull AJ, Lovett JK, Rothwell PM. Population based study of early risk of stroke after transient ischaemic attack or minor stroke: Implications for public education and organisation of services. *BMJ* 2004;**328**;326.

Table 3.1 The ABCD^2 score.

Factor	Criterion	Score
Age	60 years or over	1 point
Blood pressure	Raised on first assessment after TIA: ≥140 mmHg systolic OR ≥90 mmHg diastolic	1 point
Clinical features of TIA	Unilateral weakness of one or more of face, arm, hand or leg OR	2 points
	Speech impairment (dysarthria or dysphasia) without weakness	1 point
Duration of TIA	≥60 minutes	2 points
	10–59 minutes	1 point
Diabetes		1 point

Source: Data from Johnston SC, Rothwell PM, Nguyen-Huynh MN *et al*. Validation and refinement of scores to predict very early stroke risk after transient ischaemic attack. *Lancet* 2007;**369**:283–92.

age, blood pressure and diabetes mellitus. These risk factors have been operationalised into a simple clinical score, the ABCD^2 score, whereby people with TIA are assigned a score varying between 0 and 7, depending on the presence or absence of these features (Table 3.1). The higher the ABCD^2 score, the higher the risk of stroke (Table 3.2). About two-thirds of patients with TIA would be expected to have an ABCD^2 score ≥4, and over 90% of strokes that occur in the week following a TIA occur in patients with an ABCD^2 score ≥4.

Table 3.2 The ABCD^2 score and risk of stroke following TIA.

ABCD^2 score	Stroke risk after		
	2 days	**7 days**	**90 days**
<4	1%	1%	3%
4 or 5	4%	6%	10%
6 or 7	8%	12%	18%

Source: Data from Johnston SC, Rothwell PM, Nguyen-Huynh MN *et al.* Validation and refinement of scores to predict very early stroke risk after transient ischaemic attack. *Lancet* 2007;**369**:283–92.

Box 3.1 **NICE guideline for management of TIA**

People with a suspected TIA should receive:

- Immediate administration of aspirin
- Specialist assessment as soon as possible (within 24 hours of onset of symptoms if stroke risk high; within 1 week otherwise)
- Commencement of secondary prevention as soon as diagnosis is confirmed

Initial management of TIA

Given that about half of strokes that occur in the 90 days following a TIA occur in the first week, and that the vast majority of these occur in a sub-set of patients with distinct clinical characteristics (i.e. ABCD^2 score ≥4), it makes sense to ensure that patients are assessed urgently when a TIA occurs, and that the ABCD^2 score offers a reasonable triage tool. This is the approach that has been adopted in the English National Stroke Strategy (Figure 3.2).

Following a TIA, the first contact that most patients will have with medical services will be with their family practitioner. What should the family practitioner do?

- Consider hospital admission. This is not necessary in TIAs where the symptoms have resolved or are resolving, but will be required if a stroke rather than a TIA is suspected, due to evolution or non-resolution of symptoms.
- Assess risk of stroke using the ABCD^2 score. Use this to determine the degree of urgency with which to refer for a specialist opinion. If ABCD^2 ≥4, refer for specialist review within 24 hours (Box 3.1).
- If symptoms have resolved, initiate immediate aspirin therapy if the patient is not already on aspirin, with a loading dose of 300 mg, followed by 75 mg daily. Aspirin may be withheld by the family practitioner if symptoms have not resolved, in case the symptoms are caused by intracerebral haemorrhage (which will require brain imaging to exclude).

Investigation of a TIA

Investigations may be required to:

- Exclude alternative diagnoses
- Assess vascular risk factors
- Determine suitability for carotid endarterectomy

Alternative diagnoses

About half of referrals to specialists with a diagnosis of TIA are found to have other diagnoses. In most cases these are 'benign', such as migraine and syncope, and in many cases no clear diagnosis is made. Figure 3.3 shows diagnoses made by specialists in 317 patients referred by a general practitioner with possible TIA during the Oxford Community Stroke Project who turned out not to have a TIA. Rarer alternative diagnoses that have been made in patients referred with suspected TIA for specialist review include:

- Cerebral tumour
- Cranial nerve palsy
- Intracerebral haemorrhage
- Sub-dural haemorrhage
- Multiple sclerosis
- Cardiac arrhythmias

Assessment of vascular risk factors

Review of lifestyle, past medical history, blood pressure and serum cholesterol will help determine future vascular risk and guide strategies to reduce this risk (see Chapter 11). Specific investigations to identify possible sources of embolism include ECG (in particular looking for atrial fibrillation) and echocardiography.

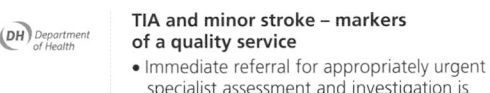

TIA and minor stroke – markers of a quality service
- Immediate referral for appropriately urgent specialist assessment and investigation is considered in all patients presenting with a recent TIA or minor stroke
- A system that identifies as urgent those with early risk of potentially preventable full stroke – to be assessed within 24 hours in high-risk cases; all other cases are assessed within seven days
- Provision to enable brain imaging within 24 hours and carotid intervention, echocardiography and ECG within 48 hours where clinically indicated
- All patients with TIA or minor stroke are followed up one month after the event, either in primary or secondary care

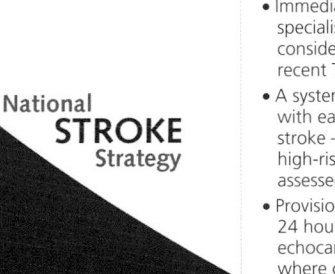

Figure 3.2 National Stroke Strategy recommendations for TIA.

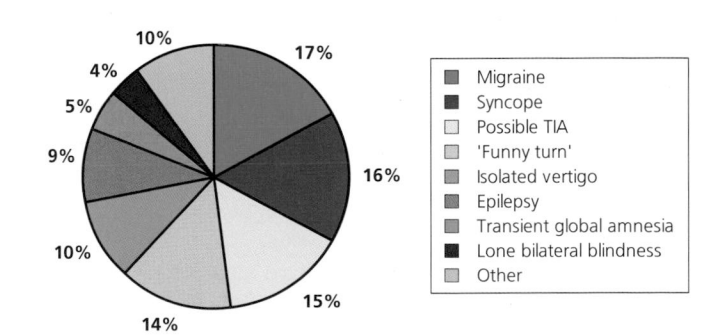

Figure 3.3 Non-TIA diagnoses made in patients referred as possible TIA. *Source*: Dennis MS, Bamford JM, Sandercock PAG, Warlow CP. Incidence of transient ischaemic attacks in Oxfordshire, England. *Stroke* 1989;**20**:333–9.

Suitability for carotid endarterectomy

People who have suffered an anterior circulation TIA or minor stroke are potential candidates for carotid endarterectomy, and therefore should have their carotid arteries assessed. Clinical signs such as carotid bruits are not reliable predictors of whether or not a patient has carotid artery stenosis. Possible ways of assessing the carotid arteries include doppler ultrasound, and MR or CT angiography.

Role of brain imaging in TIA

The role of brain imaging in acute TIA is still being established. It is important where alternative diagnoses such as cerebral tumour or intracranial haemorrhage are being considered, but this will not be the case for the majority of people presenting with symptoms suggestive of a TIA. MRI scanning with diffusion weighted imaging (DWI) is sensitive to ischaemic changes associated with TIA that will not be picked up by conventional MRI or CT scanning. This, therefore, is of particular value if the vascular territory affected by the TIA is uncertain (which will influence whether or not carotid endarterectomy should be considered; see below).

Acute pharmacological management of TIA

The following treatment strategies need to be considered:

- Antiplatelet therapy
- Anticoagulation in atrial fibrillation
- Blood pressure-lowering therapy
- Lipid-lowering therapy

The evidence from randomised controlled trials for the use of these agents in the immediate aftermath of a TIA is limited (Table 3.3). Most of the evidence (with the exception of aspirin) relates to their role in longer-term secondary prevention following a TIA.

However, promising results have been obtained from observational studies of the impact of immediate treatment of TIA, notably the EXPRESS study and the SOS-TIA study.

EXPRESS was a 'before and after' study set up to assess changes in the organisation of a daily TIA clinic in Oxford. In phase one, general practioners made urgent referrals to the clinic, where a diagnosis would be made and treatment recommendations sent back to the general practitioner. In phase two, no appointments were necessary and treatments were initiated as soon as the diagnosis had been made. The treatment regime is shown in Box 3.2. These changes were associated with:

- Reduction in the median delay to assessment in the TIA clinic from 3 days to 1 day
- Reduction in the median delay to first treatment prescription from 20 days to 1 day
- 80% reduction in risk of recurrent stroke at 90 days from 10% to 2%

In the SOS-TIA study, the impact of setting up a round-the-clock service for patients with symptoms of TIA in Paris was evaluated by comparing the actual 90-day stroke risk with that predicted from the $ABCD^2$ score. Over half of the patients were seen within 24 hours of onset of symptoms, and a stroke-prevention programme similar to that in the EXPRESS study was initiated (although dual antiplatelet therapy was not used). The expected stroke rate at 90 days was 6%,

Table 3.3 Summary of evidence from RCTs for immediate use of pharmacological agents in TIA.

Agent	Key evidence
Aspirin	Mega-trials (International Stroke Trial, IST and Chinese Acute Stroke Trial, CAST) have demonstrated an 11% reduction in risk of further vascular events if aspirin is given to people with suspected acute ischaemic stroke.
Dual antiplatelet therapy: aspirin and clopidogrel	The FASTER trial randomised 392 patients with TIA or minor stroke within 24 hours of symptom onset to aspirin +/− clopidogrel, and found a non-significant 30% reduction in risk of subsequent stroke (ischaemic or haemorrhagic) at 90 days. The MATCH trial randomised 7 599 patients within three months of a TIA or minor stroke to clopidogrel +/− aspirin. Overall, there was no evidence of benefit, and some evidence of harm in that patients receiving combination therapy had a higher risk of major haemorrhage. However, in the sub-group of patients randomised within one week of the event, there was a non-significant 17% reduction in risk of a primary event (vascular death, stroke, myocardial infarction, admission for acute ischaemia).
Dual antiplatelet therapy: aspirin and dipyridamole	No evidence for immediate use. The ESPRIT trial randomised 2 763 people within six months of a TIA or minor stroke to aspirin +/− dipyridamole and found a 20% reduction in risk of a primary event (vascular death; non-fatal stroke or myocardial infarction; or major bleed). Only 11% of participants were randomised within one week of the TIA.
Anticoagulation	No evidence for immediate use. A number of trials including over 23 000 patients have found no benefit from use of anticoagulants in acute stroke. The Warfarin–Aspirin Recurrent Stroke study (WARSS) randomised 2206 patients within one month of stroke to warfarin or aspirin and found similar risk of stroke recurrence in both groups. The European Atrial Fibrillation Trial (EAFT) randomised patients in atrial fibrillation who were within three months of a TIA or minor stroke to warfarin or aspirin, and found warfarin significantly more effective at reducing risk of recurrent stroke.
Blood pressure lowering	No evidence for immediate use. Ongoing trials are addressing the role of blood pressure lowering in acute stroke. The PROGRESS trial randomised over 6 000 people with a history of stroke or TIA and demonstrated the benefit of blood pressure lowering in this population.
Statins	The FASTER trial found no evidence of benefit of statin administration within 24 hours of a TIA or minor stroke, but the confidence intervals of the effect estimate were wide – risk ratio 1.3, 95% confidence interval 0.7–2.4).

the observed rate 1% – a similar difference in magnitude to that observed in EXPRESS.

Box 3.2 **Treatment regime in the EXPRESS study**

Loading dose of 300 mg aspirin if not already on antiplatelet therapy, followed by 75 mg daily
Loading dose of 300 mg clopidogrel, followed by 75 mg daily
Simvastatin 40 mg daily
Increase in existing blood pressure-lowering therapy, or addition of new agents if systolic blood pressure ≥130 mmHg on repeated measurement
Brain imaging was obtained for patients with incomplete resolution of symptoms to exclude intracerebral haemorrhage before giving aspirin, clopidogrel or anticoagulants (where indicated)

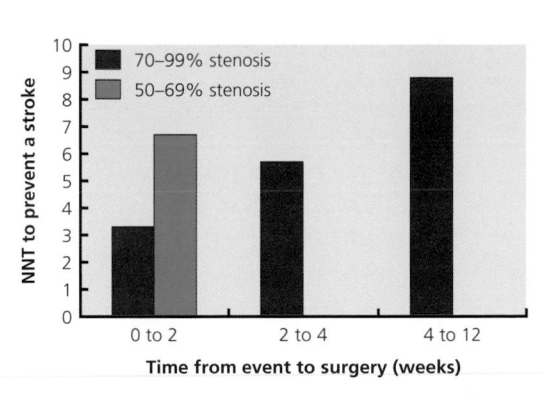

Figure 3.4 Number of carotid endarterectomies required to prevent a stroke by time from event to surgery. *Source*: Rothwell PM, Eliasziw M, Gutnikov SA, Warlow CP, Barnett HJM for the Carotid Endarterectomy Trialists Collaboration. Endarterectomy for symptomatic carotid stenosis in relation to clinical subgroups and timing of surgery. *Lancet* 2004;**363**:915–24.

The NICE guideline for acute management of TIA recommends immediate administration of aspirin, with addition of the other agents once the diagnosis has been confirmed (Box 3.1).

Role of carotid endarterectomy

Carotid endarterectomy is highly effective in reducing the risk of stroke in people who have had a recent TIA or minor stroke and have a 70% or greater stenosis in the ipsilateral carotid artery (Table 3.4).

The value of carotid endarterectomy is closely related to the timing of the surgery. Performed within two weeks, it is highly effective in reducing the risk of stroke recurrence in patients with stenosis of 50% or more (Figure 3.4). However, after two weeks it only works in people with 70% or greater stenosis, and after twelve weeks the effect is no longer statistically significant even in this group. Within the group of patients with 70% or greater stenosis, the effect tails off between two and twelve weeks: three operations will prevent one stroke in patients operated on within two weeks, but nine operations are required to prevent one stroke if the surgery is performed between four and twelve weeks after the event.

Long-term secondary prevention following TIA

The long-term risks of stroke or other vascular events remain elevated in people who have had a TIA. Therefore, longer-term management should ensure that secondary prevention strategies, both lifestyle and pharmacological, are pursued. These are discussed in Chapter 11.

Further reading

Lavallee PC, Meseguer E, Abboud H et al. A transient ischaemic attack clinic with round-the-clock access (SOS-TIA): Feasibility and effects. *Lancet Neurol* 2007;**6**:953–60.

Mant J, Wade DT, Winner S. Health care needs assessment: Stroke. In: (eds) Stevens A, Raftery J, Mant J, Simpson S. *Health Care Needs Assessment: The epidemiologically based needs assessment reviews*, First series, 2nd edn, pp 141–244. Oxford: Radcliffe Medical Press, 2004.

National Collaborating Centre for Chronic Conditions. NICE guideline for stroke – diagnosis and initial management of acute stroke and transient ischaemic attack. Royal College of Physicians, London 2008.

Pendlebury ST, Giles MF, Rothwell PM. Transient ischemic attack and stroke: diagnosis, investigation and management. Cambridge University Press, 2009.

Rothwell PM, Giles MF, Chandratheva A et al. Effect of urgent treatment of transient ischaemic attack and minor stroke on early recurrent stroke (EXPRESS study): A prospective population-based sequential comparison. *Lancet* 2007;**370**:1432–42.

Table 3.4 Impact of carotid endartertectomy by degree of symptomatic carotid stenosis.

Degree of stenosis	RR	NNT	P value
Near-occlusion	1.11	–	0.9
70–99%	0.39	6	<0.00001
50–69%	0.75	22	0.04
30–49%	0.82	31	0.6
<30%		–	0.05

Key: RR = Relative risk of ipsilateral ischaemic stroke, operative stroke or operative death over five years for surgery compared to no surgery
NNT = Number needed to treat to prevent one ipsilateral ischaemic stroke, operative stroke or operative death over five years.

Source: Rothwell PM, Eliasziw M, Gutnikov SA *et al*. for the Carotid Endarterectomy Trialists Collaboration. Analysis of pooled data from the randomised controlled trials of endarterectomy for symptomatic carotid stenosis. *Lancet* 2003;**361**:107–16.

CHAPTER 4

Acute Stroke

Damian Jenkinson and Clare Gordon

The Royal Bournemouth and Christchurch Hospitals' NHS Trust, Christchurch, UK

> **OVERVIEW**
>
> - Acute stroke is a medical emergency
> - Prehospital recognition of stroke using validated tools increases diagnostic accuracy and speed of access to hospital
> - All patients with suspected stroke should be admitted directly to a specialist acute stroke unit
> - Brain imaging is essential in acute stroke and non-contrast computerised tomography is widely available and cheap
> - Intravenous administration of recombinant tissue plasminogen activator is highly effective in selected patients

Stroke costs the UK economy £7 billion per year, and yet our clinical outcomes are poorer than in most of Europe. It seems likely that this results from differences in the way patients are managed in the acute phase of stroke. Although acute stroke is a treatable condition, it is only just beginning to be considered as a medical emergency.

Raising the public and professional profile of stroke and redesigning the acute stroke pathway to provide appropriate and effective interventions within specialist stroke services in a timely fashion will reduce mortality, morbidity and overall cost.

Urgent recognition of stroke

People with acute stroke need urgent clinical assessment and treatment. Few people have raised awareness of the symptoms of stroke, and so national campaigns are essential. The Department of Health-sponsored campaign (Figure 4.1), launched in early 2009, aimed 'to enable members of the public to recognise and identify the main symptoms of stroke, and know that it needs to be treated as an emergency'.

The campaign referenced the validated prehospital tool FAST (Face, Arm and Speech Test) to foster the public's identification of, and appropriate response to, the symptoms and signs of suspected acute stroke. FAST is used by paramedics and other health-care professionals, increasing diagnostic accuracy and speed of access to specialist care.

Within hospitals, ROSIER (Recognition of Stroke in the Emergency Room; Figure 4.2) is a more detailed assessment tool

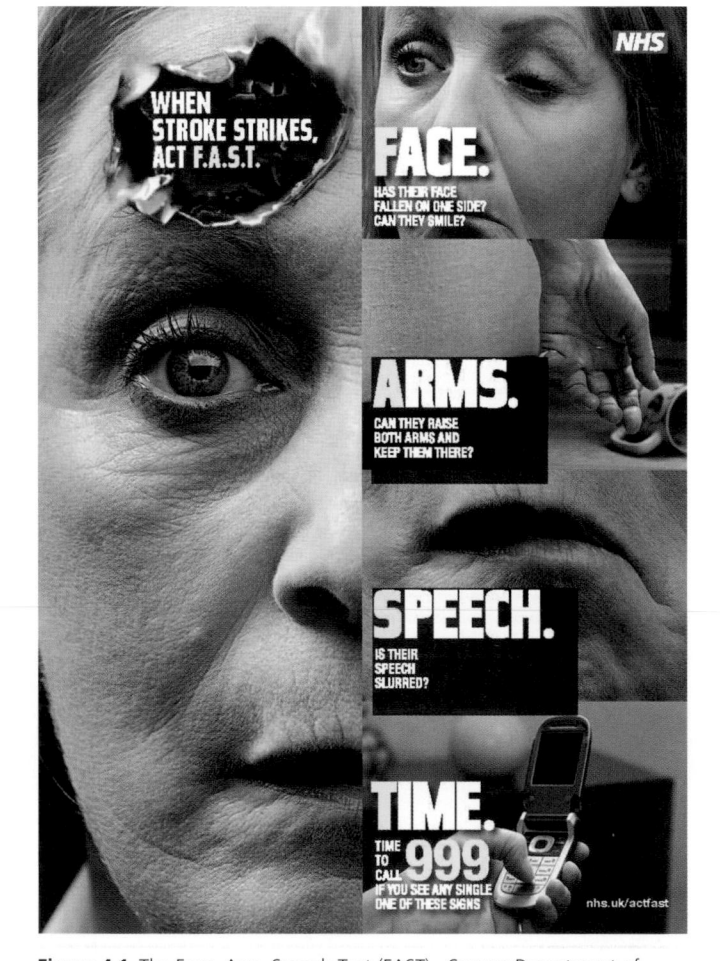

Figure 4.1 The Face, Arm, Speech Test (FAST). *Source:* Department of Health, Crown copyright 2010. Reproduced under the terms of the Click-Use Licence.

(including visual field, blood glucose and conscious level) to ensure exclusion of common stroke mimics. The four 'Ss' – seizure, syncope, sepsis and somatisation – account for two-thirds of stroke mimics (Table 4.1).

Immediate assessment

Initial assessment of all patients with acute stroke should take place within a specialist acute stroke service. Triage of patients with suspected acute stroke to such a facility should be undertaken

ABC of Stroke. Edited by Jonathan Mant and Marion F Walker.
© 2011 Blackwell Publishing Ltd.

Glasgow Coma Scale: Eyes =   Motor =   Verbal =

BP =   *BM =

* If BM < 3.5 mmol/ltreat urgently and reassess once blood glucose normal

1. Has there been loss of consciousness or syncope?

                                    Y(–1) ☐   N(0) ☐

2. Has there been seizure activity?

                                    Y(–1) ☐   N(0) ☐

3. Is there a <u>NEW ACUTE</u> onset or on awakening from sleep

Asymmetric facial weakness	Y(1) ☐	N(0) ☐
Asymmetric grip weakness	Y(1) ☐	N(0) ☐
Asymmetric arm weakness	Y(1) ☐	N(0) ☐
Asymmetric leg weakness	Y(1) ☐	N(0) ☐
Speech disturbance	Y(1) ☐	N(0) ☐
Visual field defect	Y(1) ☐	N(0) ☐

                        ** Total Score _____ (–2 to +6)

**Admit to Acute Stroke Unit / Refer to stroke team if total score > 0 (score between 1 and 6)

Figure 4.2 ROSIER (Recognition of Stroke in the Emergency Room).

Table 4.1 Stroke mimics.

Seizures	24%
Syncope	23%
Sepsis	10%
Somatisation	7%
Migraine	6%
Labyrinthitis	4%
Brain tumour	3%
Hypoglycaemia	3%
Others	20%

with the same priority as patients with acute myocardial infarction. For patients presenting within three hours of stroke onset, it is particularly important that thrombolysis is considered, and that early assessment is performed as rapidly as possible. Evaluation comprises:

1 Immediate cardiorespiratory condition, including:
   ○ Airway
   ○ Breathing
   ○ Circulation
2 History
   ○ Confirmation of diagnosis of stroke
   ○ Clarification of onset time and presentation with witnesses/paramedics
   ○ Past medical history, current medications and risk factors for stroke
   ○ Prestroke function/level of disability
   ○ Standard disability measures are useful to communicate level of disability and provide structure to the assessment; commonly used disability measures include the Barthel Score and the Modified Rankin Score (Tables 4.2 and 4.3)
3 General physical examination: body temperature and pulse oximetry should be taken. Cardiovascular examination focuses on current or recent myocardial ischaemia, rhythm and valvular abnormalities, aortic dissection and embolic manifestations.
4 Neurological examination: assessment of current stroke severity is best done using a formal stroke scale. Most commonly used is the National Institute of Health Stroke Scale (Table 4.4).

Investigation

Brain imaging

Brain imaging is essential in acute stroke to exclude haemorrhage and stroke mimics. Non-contrast computerised tomography

Table 4.2 Barthel score.

Activity	Description	Score
1 Urinary continence	Fully continent	2
	Incontinent less than once a day	1
	Incontinent more than once a day, or catheterised	0
2 Faecal continence	Continent	2
	Incontinent less than once a week	1
	Incontinent more than once a week, or requires enema	0
3 Grooming (face/hair/teeth/shaving)	Independent (implements provided)	1
	Needs help	0
4 Toilet use	Independent (including clothes and wiping)	2
	Needs some help	1
	Dependent	0
5 Feeding	Independent (feed provided within reach)	2
	Needs help (cutting up food, spreading butter)	1
	Unable	0
6 Transfer	Independent	3
	Minor help (prompting or assistance of one)	2
	Major help	1
	Unable	0
7 Mobility	Independent (with/without aid)	3
	Walks with help of one person (verbal/physical)	2
	Wheelchair independent	1
	Unable	0
8 Dressing	Independent (including buttons, zips, laces)	2
	Needs help but can do half unaided	1
	Dependent	0
9 Stairs	Independent up and down	2
	Needs help (verbal/physical/carrying aid)	1
	Unable	0
10 Bathing	Independent bathing or showering	1
	Dependent	0
Barthel score (out of 20)		

Table 4.3 Modified Rankin Scale.

Score	Description
0	No symptoms at all
1	No significant disability despite symptoms; able to carry out all usual duties and activities
2	Slight disability; unable to carry out all previous activities, but able to look after own affairs without assistance
3	Moderate disability; requiring some help, but able to walk without assistance
4	Moderately severe disability; unable to walk without assistance and unable to attend to own bodily needs without assistance
5	Severe disability; bedridden, incontinent and requiring constant nursing care and attention
6	Dead

Table 4.4 National Institute of Health Stroke Scale.

Tested Item	Title	Responses and Scores
1A	Level of consciousness	0 – alert 1 – drowsy 2 – obtunded 3 – coma/unresponsive
1B	Orientation questions (2)	0 – answers both correctly 1 – answers one correctly 2 – answers neither correctly
1C	Response to commands (2)	0 – performs both tasks correctly 1 – performs one task correctly 2 – performs neither
2	Gaze	0 – normal horizontal movements 1 – partial gaze palsy 2 – complete gaze palsy
3	Visual fields	0 – no visual field defect 1 – partial hemianopia 2 – complete hemianopia 3 – bilateral hemianopia
4	Facial movement	0 – normal 1 – minor facial weakness 2 – partial facial weakness 3 – complete unilateral palsy
5	Motor function (arm) **a.** Left **b.** Right	0 – no drift 1 – drift before 5 seconds 2 – falls before 10 seconds 3 – no effort against gravity 4 – no movement
6	Motor function (leg) **a.** Left **b.** Right	0 – no drift 1 – drift before 5 seconds 2 – falls before 5 seconds 3 – no effort against gravity 4 – no movement
7	Limb ataxia	0 – no ataxia 1 – ataxia in 1 limb 2 – ataxia in 2 limbs
8	Sensory	0 – no sensory loss 1 – mild sensory loss 2 – severe sensory loss
9	Language	0 – normal 1 – mild aphasia 2 – severe aphasia 3 – mute or global aphasia
10	Articulation	0 – normal 1 – mild dysarthria 2 – severe dysarthria
11	Extinction or inattention	0 – absent 1 – mild (loss 1 sensory modality) 2 – severe (loss 2 modalities)

(NCCT) has the advantages that it is widely available and cheap, is sensitive to haemorrhage and has a rapid acquisition time. Its disadvantages are the radiation used, low sensitivity (<50% within 5 h) to hyperacute infarction, inability to identify hypoperfused but viable brain and poor imaging of the posterior fossa.

Interpretation of NCCT should be structured to systematically exclude intracerebral haemorrhage and other intracranial lesions, and to exclude early signs of major ischaemia that are associated with increased risk of haemorrhage when using thrombolysis. This includes the presence of sulcal effacement and blurring of grey-white junction in more than one third of the territory of the middle cerebral artery. A scaling system such as ASPECTS (Alberta Stroke Program Early CT Score; Figure 4.3) can facilitate this assessment.

Other brain-imaging modalities have advantages over NCCT but are currently far less available. Multi-modal magnetic resonance imaging (MRI) can reveal the extent of ischaemic injury (DWI, diffusion weighted imaging), demonstrate perfusion status (PWI, perfusion weighted imaging), estimate the presence and extent of the ischaemic penumbra, reveal vessel status with angiography, and identify haemorrhage with gradient echo. Perfusion computerised tomography (PCT; see Figure 4.4) is an evolving technology offering similar advantages to multi-modal MRI.

Brain imaging should be performed immediately (definitely within one hour) for people with acute stroke who have any of the following: indications for thrombolysis, taking anticoagulants, known bleeding tendency, a depressed level of consciousness, progressive or fluctuating symptoms, papilloedema, neck stiffness or fever, or severe headache at onset of stroke. For all other people with acute stroke, imaging should be performed within a maximum of 24 hours of onset of symptoms.

Diagnostic tests

Electrocardiography should be performed in all stroke patients, as myocardial infarction can lead to stroke, and arrhythmias, particularly atrial fibrillation, are common. Blood sugar, full blood count, biochemistry, erythrocyte sedimentation rate and clotting (ordered urgently if thrombolysis considered) exclude stroke mimics and influence management.

Selected patients should undergo chest radiography (if lung disease or heart failure is suspected), arterial blood gas analysis, lumbar puncture (if sub-arachnoid haemorrhage is suspected and CT scan is negative for blood) and drug toxicology.

Monitoring and stabilisation

Stroke unit care

People with suspected acute stroke should be admitted directly to a specialist acute stroke unit for monitoring and stabilisation;

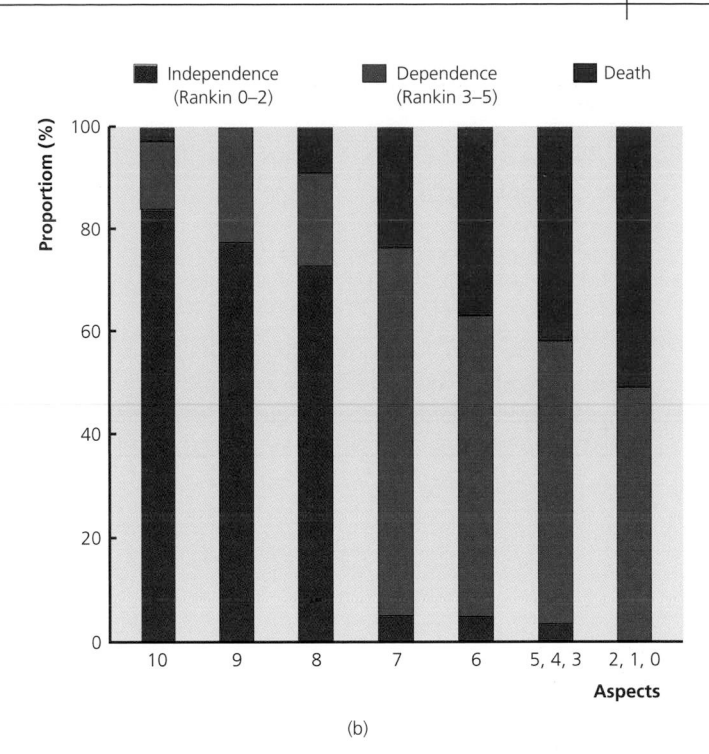

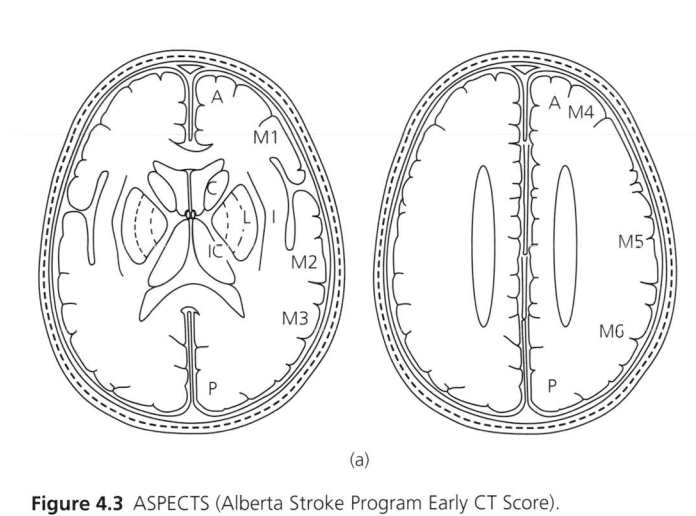

(a)

(b)

Figure 4.3 ASPECTS (Alberta Stroke Program Early CT Score).
One point is allocated for each of 10 specified areas on the non-contrast CT scan that does not show early ischaemic changes. The total score, between 0 and 10, correlates with the clinical outcomes of the patient, with a score of < 7 predicting very poor outcome and increased likelihood of haemorrhage with thrombolytic therapy. *Source:* From Barber *et al.*, 2000, and 2004, with permission.

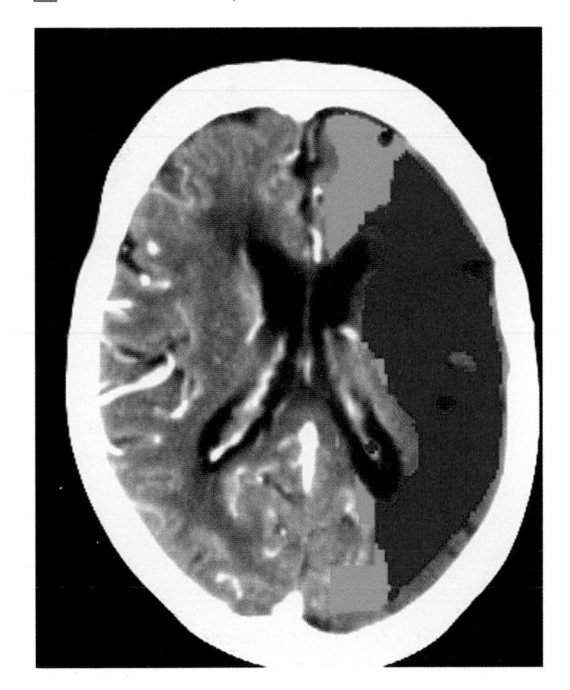

Figure 4.4 Perfusion CT in acute stroke.

this is guidance from the National Institute of Health and Clinical Excellence (NICE) 2008. Patients admitted to organised stroke care are less likely to die and more likely to leave hospital independent than are those cared for on general medical wards. 49% of UK Trusts have an acute stroke unit, characterised by access to brain imaging within 24 hours, specialist ward rounds at least five times a week, and acute stroke protocols and guidelines. A significant proportion also have access to CT scanning within three hours, continuous physiological monitoring and policies for direct admission from the Emergency Room.

Protocols on an acute stroke unit should exist for detection and management in the following areas:

- Swallow screen on admission
- Cognition and communication screening
- Urinalysis and continence assessment
- Nutrition assessment (including weight)
- Falls risk assessment
- Pressure ulcer risk assessment

Maintaining homeostasis

The following are based on recommendations from NICE guidance (2008):

- *Supplementary oxygen*: Supplementary oxygen is not recommended for people with acute stroke who are not hypoxic. Oxygen should be administered if oxygen saturation drops below 95%.
- *Blood sugar*: People with acute stroke should be treated to maintain a blood glucose between 4 and 11 mmol/litre. Optimal insulin therapy should be provided to all adults with diabetes who have threatened or actual acute myocardial infarction or stroke.
- *Blood pressure*: Manipulation of blood pressure after acute stroke is not recommended except where there is evidence of hypertensive encephalopathy, nephropathy, heart failure or myocardial infarction, evidence of aortic dissection, pre-eclampsia/

eclampsia, or intracerebral haemorrhage with systolic blood pressure above 200 mmHg.

- *Hydration and nutrition*: Routine nutritional supplementation is not recommended for people with acute stroke who are adequately nourished. People with acute stroke who are unable to take adequate nutrition and fluids orally should receive early (within 24 hours of admission) feeding through a nasogastric tube.

Treatment

Early mobilisation and rehabilitation

People with acute stroke should be mobilised as soon as possible, after an assessment (including sitting balance and falls risk) by an appropriately trained health-care professional, with access to appropriate equipment. Even if the patient is too unwell for active rehabilitation, a 24-hour therapeutic approach should be adopted by the nursing team, who will be providing the most patient input in the acute phase.

Thrombolysis

Intravenous administration of recombinant tissue plasminogen activator (r-tPA) is recommended by NICE for the treatment of acute ischaemic stroke within three hours of onset, when used by physicians trained and experienced in the management of acute stroke. Characteristics of patients with ischaemic stroke who could be treated with r-tPA are shown in Table 4.5. It should only be administered within a well-organised stroke service, and protocols should be in place for the delivery and management of thrombolysis, including postthrombolysis complications.

The trial ECASS (European Cooperative Acute Stroke Study) III has confirmed continuing efficacy of r-tPA within the 3- to 4.5-hour

Table 4.5 Characteristics of patients with ischaemic stroke who could be treated with r-tPA.

Diagnosis of ischemic stroke causing measurable neurological deficit.
The neurological signs should not be clearing spontaneously.
The neurological signs should not be minor and isolated.
Caution should be exercised in treating a patient with major deficits.
The symptoms of stroke should not be suggestive of subarachnoid hemorrhage.
Onset of symptoms <3 hours before beginning treatment
No head trauma or prior stroke in previous 3 months
No myocardial infarction in the previous 3 months
No gastrointestinal or urinary tract hemorrhage in previous 21 days
No major surgery in the previous 14 days
No arterial puncture at a noncompressible site in the previous 7 days
No history of previous intracranial hemorrhage
Blood pressure not elevated (systolic <185 mmHg and diastolic <110 mmHg)
No evidence of active bleeding or acute trauma (fracture) on examination
Not taking an oral anticoagulant or, if anticoagulant being taken, INR ≤ 1.7
If receiving heparin in previous 48 hours, aPTT must be in normal range.
Platelet count ≥100 000 mm³
Blood glucose concentration ≥50 mg/dL (2.7 mmol/L)
No seizure with postictal residual neurological impairments
CT does not show a multilobar infarction (hypodensity >1/3 cerebral hemisphere).
The patient or family members understand the potential risks and benefits from treatment.

INR indicates international normalized ratio; aPTT, activated partial thromboplastin time.

window, but these data have not as yet been incorporated into the NIICE guidance, nor has the drug licence been extended beyond 3 hours.

Intra-arterial thrombolysis is an option for the treatment of highly selected patients who have major stroke of less than 6 hours duration, and who are not otherwise candidates for intravenous r-tPA. Treatment requires the patient to be at an experienced stroke centre with immediate access to cerebral angiography and qualified interventional neuroradiologists.

Antiplatelet treatment

All people with acute stroke, who have had a diagnosis of primary intracerebral haemorrhage excluded by brain imaging, should receive aspirin 300 mg no later than 24 hours after stroke. Thereafter, aspirin 300 mg should be continued until two weeks after stroke, at which time long-term secondary prevention antiplatelet therapy should be prescribed.

Statin therapy

People with ischaemic stroke and total cholesterol of 3.5 mmol/l or greater should be initiated on a statin prior to discharge. Immediate initiation of statin following acute stroke is not recommended because of the potential increased risk of haemorrhagic transformation. Patients with ischaemic stroke who are already taking a statin should continue the therapy.

Surgery for acute intracerebral haemorrhage

Surgery is rarely required for people with small, deep haemorrhage, lobar haemorrhage without hydrocephalus, large haemorrhage and significant comorbidities, or a GCS less than 8. Previously fit people should be considered for surgery if there is lobar haemorrhage with hydrocephalus, or they are deteriorating neurologically.

Patients with cerebellar haematoma are at particular risk of deterioration through compression of the brain stem and hydrocephalus. The consensus is that such patients should be referred to neurosurgical specialists for consideration of evacuation of haematoma.

Surgery for decompressive hemicraniectomy

People with middle cerebral artery (MCA) infarction complicated by massive brain oedema (malignant MCA syndrome) have a mortality rate of 80%, and selected patients will benefit from decompressive hemicraniectomy. Suitable patients are aged up to 60 years, referred within 24 hours of onset, treated within 48 hours, and have clinical and radiographic evidence of MCA territory infarction, with a decrease in conscious level.

End-of-life care

The risk of dying in the first seven days after a stroke is around 12%, and early clinical signs of severe brainstem dysfunction are highly predictive of death. In the first days after stroke, most patients die as a result of the stroke itself. If they survive the first days, the main risk of death is then from complications of the stroke, such as pneumonia or pulmonary embolus.

If after the initial assessment the management decision is palliative care, this decision should be reviewed on a daily basis by the stroke team. The patient should still have access to stroke unit care. If death is considered to be imminent, then a palliative care pathway, such as the Liverpool Care Pathway, can provide guidance on symptom management.

Further reading

American Heart Association/American Stroke Association. Guidelines for the early management of adults with ischemic stroke. *Stroke* 2007;**38**: 1655–1711.

Department of Health. *National Stroke Strategy*. London: Department of Health, 2007.

National Collaborating Centre for Chronic Conditions. *Stroke: Diagnosis and initial management of acute stroke and transient ischaemic attack (TIA)*. London: National Collaborating Centre for Chronic Conditions, 2008.

Royal College of Physicians. *National Clinical Guidelines for Stroke*, 3rd edn. London: Royal College of Physicians, 2008.

CHAPTER 5

Medical Complications of Stroke

Clare Gordon and Damian Jenkinson

The Royal Bournemouth and Christchurch Hospitals' NHS Trust, Christchurch, UK

OVERVIEW

- Patients with stroke are at high risk of developing medical complications
- Such complications impede rehabilitation, are associated with poor functional outcome and increase costs
- Awareness of potential complications and a systematic approach to identifying and managing them are key elements of an organised stroke service

---

Medical complications after stroke are common, present barriers to optimal recovery, are related to poor outcomes and are potentially preventable or treatable. Estimates of frequency of complications range from 40% to 96% of patients, with severity of stroke being the most important risk factor.

Rigorous attention to detail in the prevention and treatment of complications should improve stroke outcomes. The data from the randomised trials of stroke unit care indicate that the causes of death that are most likely to be prevented by stroke unit care are those classified as complications of immobility (in particular, thromboembolism and infection).

Classification and frequency of complications

A simple clinical classification of complications of stroke and the frequency of symptomatic complications, from a prospective multi-centre study, is shown in Table 5.1. There are high frequencies of infections (urinary tract infection, chest infection and other types of infection causing pyrexial illness), pressure sores, falls, pain other than shoulder pain and confusion.

Most complications develop within the first six weeks after stroke (Figure 5.1), with an early onset being seen particularly for pressure sores, pain and infections. Falls and depression appear to develop more gradually, perhaps reflecting progress in rehabilitation (falls) or a reluctance to make an early diagnosis of depression.

ABC of Stroke. Edited by Jonathan Mant and Marion F Walker.
© 2011 Blackwell Publishing Ltd.

Table 5.1 Frequency of symptomatic complications in hospitalised stroke patients.

Complication	Frequency, % (95% CI)
Neurological	
Recurrent stroke	9 (6–12)
Epileptic seizure	3 (1–5)
Infections	
Urinary tract infection	23 (18–28)
Chest infection	22 (18–27)
Other infection	19 (15–24)
Mobility	
Pressure sore/skin break	21 (16–25)
Fall, serious injury	5 (2–7)
Fall, no injury	21 (16–25)
Fall, total	25 (21–30)
Thromboembolism	
Deep vein thrombosis	2 (0–3)
Pulmonary embolism	1 (0–2)
Pain	
Shoulder pain	9 (6–12)
Other pain	34 (28–39)
Psychological	
Depression	16 (12–21)
Emotionalism	12 (8–15)
Anxiety	14 (10–18)
Confusion	36 (30–41)
Miscellaneous	61 (55–66)

Source: Adapted from Langhorne P, Stott DJ, Robertson L *et al.* Medical complications after stroke: A multicenter study. *Stroke* 2000;**31**(6):1223–9.

Infection after stroke

Poststroke infection (PSI) occurs in around 25–65% of patients admitted with aute stroke to hospital, with urinary tract infection (UTI) and chest infection being the most frequent (Table 5.1).

Predisposing factors for developing PSI after stroke include dysphagia, urinary incontinence (and urinary catheterisation) and reduced level of consciousness. Approximately half of all stroke patients with dysphagia experience aspiration, and over a third of these patients develop aspiration pneumonia. Nasogastric feeding provides only limited protection against aspiration pneumonia. Urinary catheterisation increases the odds of developing a poststroke UTI by three- to fourfold.

PSI is associated with poor short-term outcomes, including in-hospital death, functional recovery and institutionalisation on

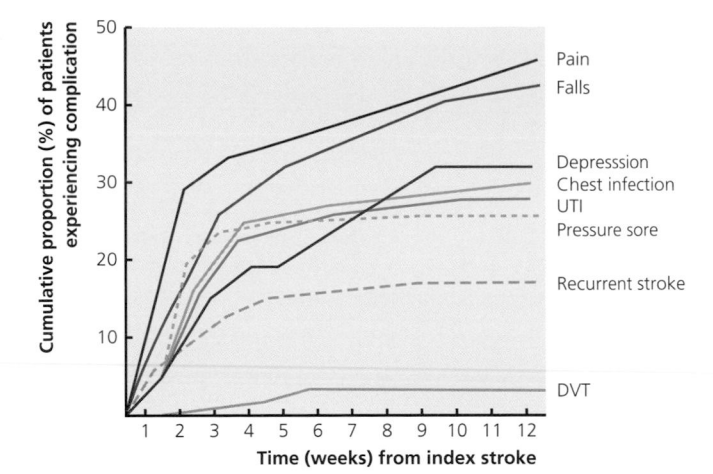

Figure 5.1 Timing of symptomatic complications after stroke. *Source:* Langhorne P, Stott DJ, Robertson L *et al. Medical complications after stroke: A multicenter study. Stroke* 2000;**31**(6):1223–9. Reproduced with permission from Wolters Kluwer Health.

discharge; and these associations are independent of stroke severity, age and prestroke level of independence. The effects of PSI on longer-term outcomes are virtually unknown.

The most important aspect of managing PSI is a low threshold for suspecting a diagnosis. However, non-septic fever can be misinterpreted as PSI (and inappropriately treated with antibiotics) if physical examination fails to reveal clear focal signs of infection and if the necessary investigations are not undertaken to confirm the presence of bacteria.

Organised stroke unit care facilitates early detection and treatment of PSI. The mainstay of specific treatment of PSI is appropriate antibiotic therapy. Limited data suggest that prophylactic antibiotic therapy is not beneficial. Many other aspects of patient care – such as patient positioning or the use of thickened fluids – that may potentially be important in preventing PSI have not undergone formal evaluation. It is well recognised that avoiding use of indwelling urinary catheters will significantly reduce urinary PSI.

Reduced mobility after stroke

Immobility-related complications are very common in the first year after a stroke and low Barthel scores correlate with a high number of complications. The major immobility-related complications are pressure ulcers, venous thromboembolism, pain and falls.

Pressure ulcers

Pressure ulcers can occur anywhere on the body, but are most common over bony prominences. The incidence of pressure ulcers for inpatients with stroke is 21%, as compared with the national incidence for all inpatients of 4–10%. The risk factors for pressure ulcers commonly found in stroke patients are listed in Table 5.2.

Assessment is required within six hours of admission. Risk assessment tools, such as the Norton or Waterlow scores, can be used, but should not replace clinical judgement.

Early mobilisation is the key to prevention of pressure ulcers, and should be part of the patient's rehabilitation plan. The choice of

Table 5.2 Risk factors for developing pressure ulcers.

Reduced mobility	Sensory impairment
Acute illness	Reduced level of consciousness
Greater than 65 years of age	Vascular disease
Malnutrition and dehydration	Severe chronic illness

Source: Adapted from Royal College of Nursing. *Pressure Ulcer Risk Assessment and Prevention: Recommendations 2001.* London: RCN, 2001.

Table 5.3 A summary of the benefits of pressure-relieving interventions.

Level of benefit	Type of intervention	References
Beneficial	Alternative foam mattresses compared to standard hospital mattresses	Cullum *et al.* (2004)
Likely	Regular repositioning (expert consensus)	
	Alternating pressure mattresses Silicone or foam overlays	Cullum *et al.* (2004)
Unknown	Kinetic turning tables Seat cushions	Cullum *et al.* (2004)
	Dietary supplementation	Langer *et al.* (2003)
No benefit	Water-filled gloves Sheepskins (synthetic or real)	Cullum *et al.* (2004)
	Doughnut-shaped cushions/rings Foot waffle heel elevators	NICE (2001)

Sources: Cullum N, McInnes E, Bell-Sayer SEM, Legood R. Support surfaces for pressure ulcer prevention. *Cochrane Database of Systematic Reviews* 2004, Issue 3. NICE. *Pressure Ulcer Risk Assessment and Prevention.* London: National Institute for Health and Clinical Excellence, 2001. Langer G, Schloemer G, Knerr A, Kuss O, Behrens J. Nutritional interventions for preventing and treating pressure ulcers. *Cochrane Database of Systematic Reviews* 2003, Issue 4.

pressure-relieving aid (Table 5.3) should not only be based on level of risk but patient comfort, positioning and rehabilitation needs. All patients with a risk of pressure ulcers should be placed on a minimum of a high-specification foam mattress.

Venous thromboembolism

The reported frequency of deep vein thrombosis (DVT) after stroke may be as high as 50% of patients with hemiplegia, but the rate of symptomatic pulmonary embolism is low, ranging from 1% to 7%.

Clinical signs of DVT can be difficult to assess after stroke due to impaired consciousness, dysphasia, inattention, dependent oedema and reduced sensation. Symptoms and signs, if present, may include a swollen, hot or painful limb, and fever.

Measures to help prevent DVT should include early mobilisation and adequate hydration and nutrition. Aspirin should be prescribed to those patients where cerebral haemorrhage has been excluded by brain imaging. Prophylactic heparin should not routinely be used, and should only be used in selected high-risk patients. A large randomised controlled trial has demonstrated that full-length graduated compression stockings do not reduce the risk of symptomatic or asymptomatic DVT after stroke, when compared with best medical care only.

If a DVT is suspected, the first-line investigation is Doppler ultrasound. After ischaemic stroke, patients with a proven DVT should be anticoagulated – in preference to treatment with aspirin – unless contraindicated. There is an absence of evidence to guide treatment of DVT after haemorrhagic stroke, but the consensus is that patients should either receive antiplatelet therapy or have a vena-caval filter inserted.

Stroke-related pain

Many patients will develop some form of pain after their stroke. This may be due to pre-existing conditions, such as osteoarthritis, or neuropathic or shoulder pain as a result of the stroke. Every patient should be routinely asked if they have any pain and its severity. Correct positioning with mobilisation can help prevent shoulder and musculosketetal pain.

Poststroke pain syndrome typically follows thalamic or medullary infarctions. Treatment for neuropathic and poststroke pain is similar, and should be treated with one or more of antidepressants and anticonvulsants. If the pain is poorly controlled, the patient should be referred to a specialist in pain management.

Shoulder pain may have a number of contributing factors. Weakness of shoulder girdle muscles increases the risk of subluxation and pain. The shoulder should be supported and kept in alignment at all times to prevent damage and pain, and to reinforce normal movement principles.

Adhesive capsulitis may result from paralysis, and while slings and immobilising devices may make the patient feel more secure, there is no evidence that they improve outcome.

Falls

In one study on an acute stroke unit, non-serious falls occurred in 21% of unselected stroke inpatients, and serious falls (resulting in bone fracture, or head and soft tissue injury) in less than 5%. Falls are frequent among patients who are dependent in activities of daily living, with 79% of such people falling in the first six months at home.

It is important to use recognised scaling systems to systematically identify patients who are at particular risk of falling. Patients should be mobilised with adequate supervision by a multidisciplinary team in an appropriately lit environment. Withdrawal of unnecessary drugs may be useful.

Neurological complications after stroke

About 25% of patients with acute stroke have neurological deterioration within the first 48 hours and, of these, the most important neurological causes are:

- Progressive or recurrent stroke (one third of patients)
- Ischaemic brain swelling (one third)
- Haemorrhagic transformation of an infarct (10%)
- Seizure (10%)

Recurrent stroke

Using the definition of recurrent stroke as neurological deterioration after 24 hours or more after the incident event, involving any vascular territory, the 90-day risk of recurrent stroke is around 18%. In the long term, the annual stroke risk remains at about nine times the risk of stroke in the general population of the same age and sex.

Effective secondary prevention measures (see Chapter 11) should be started as soon as possible after stroke, and probably continue over life.

Ischaemic brain swelling

The risk of symptomatic brain swelling in patients with anterior circulation ischaemic stroke is estimated to be 10% to 20%, and the incidence in posterior stroke is unknown. Brain swelling most typically occurs in patients with occlusion of the stem of the middle cerebral artery (MCA), appearing about four days after stroke onset. The term 'malignant MCA syndrome' has been used to delineate patients with large territorial infarcts that swell within 24 hours, causing brain herniation signs.

Few clinical signs predict deterioration, but the need for early mechanical ventilation increases the risk of death. Factors that exacerbate swelling, such as hypoxia, hypercapnia and hyperthermia, should probably be corrected. Decompressive hemicraniectomy is indicated in selected patients with malignant MCA syndrome (see Chapter 4) and management of cerebellar swelling should include decompressive suboccipital craniotomy.

Haemorrhagic transformation of infarct

While post-mortem series suggest that almost all infarctions have some element of petechial bleeding, prospective studies using CT brain scanning estimate a rate of haemorrhagic transformation of about 5%. Small asymptomatic petechiae are much less important than haematomas, which may be associated with neurological decline. The use of anticoagulants and thrombolytics increases the risk of serious haemorrhagic transformation, but must be weighed against the benefits of these agents.

Management of patients with haemorrhagic transformation of infarct depends on the amount of bleeding and symptoms, and clot evacuation may be appropriate in deteriorating patients. Haemorrhagic transformation in patients with cerebellar infarction significantly increases the risk of deterioration. Functional outcome in patients with haemorrhagic transformation on CT scanning admitted to rehabilitation is not significantly different from patients without such changes.

Seizures

Poststroke seizures within the first 24 hours after stroke onset occur in 2% to 33% of patients, and the late seizure rate ranges from 3% to 67%. The risk of late seizures is higher in people with pre-existing dementia.

Status epilepticus is uncommon, but continuing partial seizure activity should be considered in patients after stroke who deteriorate or fail to recover at an anticipated rate. Recommendations on the use of individual anticonvulsants are based on the established management of seizures complicating any neurological illness.

Continence and constipation after stroke

Urinary incontinence

Between 32% and 79% of stroke patients are incontinent immediately after stroke. Incontinence is associated with increased morbidity and mortality, carer strain and institutionalisation, and is linked with stroke severity. At six months, 20% of stroke patients will still have incontinence. All patients with a stroke should receive an initial assessment on admission, mainly to exclude retention and infection (Table 5.4). If at two weeks the incontinence persists, further assessments and a management plan should be initiated.

Treatment is dictated by the underlying cause of the incontinence. For urge incontinence, suggested by symptoms of frequency and urgency, bladder training and reducing caffeine intake are appropriate. Antimuscarinic drugs should only be considered if retention is excluded. The first-line treatment for stress incontinence or mixed symptoms is pelvic floor exercises.

Retention or incomplete emptying is suggested by symptoms of a residual volume >100 ml, recurrent infections and constant dribbling. It is important that constipation is excluded. In acute urinary retention, patients may require catheterisation while further assessments of the cause of retention are undertaken. The catheter should be removed as soon as possible.

Functional incontinence is treated by reducing the impact of the patient's disability. This includes improving mobility, loose clothing for quick access and ensuring a call bell and picture cards (if appropriate) are available. Alternative strategies while immobile include urinals for both male and female.

Faecal incontinence and constipation

Bowel dysfunction is common after stroke, with up to 40% affected by faecal incontinence and up to 60% with constipation.

Assessment is outlined in Table 5.5. Most bowel dysfunction can be improved by resolving faecal loading (assessed by rectal examination or abdominal x-ray) and treating infective diarrhoea.

Table 5.4 Urinary assessment after stroke.

Longstanding/new symptoms of incontinence	Ideally 3 days' frequency and volume chart
Drug history	Check for constipation, rectal examination
Obstetric/prostatic problems	Postvoid residual urine volume
Urinalysis (for glucose, protein, blood and leucocytes and nitrites)	MSU if urinalysis shows positive for leucocytes and nitrites
Cognition and communication	

Table 5.5 Faecal continence assessment after stroke.

Normal bowel habit and current pattern	Stool chart, e.g. Bristol Stool Chart
Drug history	Rectal examination
Awareness of need to defaecate/level of consciousness	Mobility and toileting facilities (e.g. bed pan/commode/toilet)
Cognition and communication	Potentially treatable causes of diarrhoea (e.g. infective, irritable bowel syndrome)

Swallowing, nutrition and hydration

Swallowing

Around half of all patients admitted with stroke are unable to swallow initially, and most of these will recover their swallow within a month. Swallowing difficulties put the patient at risk of aspiration, malnutrition and dehydration. Most patients who survive with dysphagia will improve within a few weeks.

All patients should receive a swallow screen on admission to determine if they have a safe swallow. If they have an unsafe swallow, they should be kept nil by mouth until a specialist assessment of swallowing has been performed. Plans for hydration, nutrition (within 48 hours) and regular mouth care should be made while waiting for specialist assessments.

Nutrition

All patients need their nutritional status and risk of malnutrition assessed on admission along with their ability to swallow. This should include a weight and Body Mass Index calculation.

If the patient is able to swallow, it is important that they are assisted with their feeding, depending on their level of disability. Documentation of their nutritional intake along with regular nutritional assessments will inform the team if the patient is taking adequate amounts. Some patients with inadequate intake can be supplemented with nasogastric (NG) feeding. Routine oral dietary supplementation has been proven not to be beneficial.

Dysphagia should be managed by either a modified consistency diet or NG feeding, depending on the specialist assessment. People with acute stroke who are unable to take adequate nutrition and fluids orally should:

- receive tube feeding with an NG tube within 24 hours of admission;
- be considered for a nasal bridle tube or gastrostomy if they are unable to tolerate an NG tube.

Often deciding to commence enteral feeding is a difficult decision, and the multi-disciplinary team should consider the patient's prognosis, co-morbidities, capacity and ability to consent. If the patient is unable to consent for themselves, it is good practice to try to ascertain the patient's wishes from their next of kin.

All attempts at NG feeding should be exhausted (including a nasal bridle for recurrent removals) before an early gastrostomy tube is inserted, due to the increased risks of death and poor outcome with early gastrostomy insertion.

Hydration

Dehydration is usually caused by inadequate intake due to reduced level of consciousness, reliance on others to provide drinks, reduced sensitivity to thirst, dysphagia or infection. It can theoretically worsen cerebral ischaemia through a drop in blood pressure and raised haematocrit, and increases the risk of venous thromboembolism.

Daily haematocrit, urea and electrolytes should be monitored in the acute phase, as these are more sensitive indicators than clinical signs of dehydration.

Patients unable to take adequate oral fluids need supplementation by either intravenous, subcutaneous or nasogastric routes.

Further reading

Department of Health. *National Stroke Strategy*. London: Department of Health, 2007.

National Institute for Health and Clinical Excellence. *Pressure Ulcer Risk Assessment and Prevention (Guideline B)*. London: NICE, 2001.

National Institute for Health and Clinical Excellence. *Nutritional Support in Adults: Oral nutrition support, enteral tube feeding and parenteral nutrition*. London: NICE, 2006.

National Institute for Health and Clinical Excellence. *Urinary Incontinence: The management of urinary incontinence in women*. London: NICE, 2006.

National Institute for Health and Clinical Excellence. *Faecal Incontinence: The management of faecal incontinence in adults*. London: NICE, 2007.

Royal College of Physicians. *National Clinical Guidelines for Stroke*, 3rd edn. London: Royal College of Physicians, 2008.

CHAPTER 6

Stroke Rehabilitation

Marion F Walker

University of Nottingham, Nottingham, UK

OVERVIEW

- All patients who have activity limitations should receive stroke rehabilitation intervention regardless of stroke severity

- Multi-disciplinary assessment should be continuous and findings should be communicated regularly to all team members

- Early Supported Discharge teams reduce time spent in hospital and can facilitate functional recovery in mild to moderate stroke patients

- Patients should receive as much rehabilitation as they can tolerate

- Where possible patients should be offered rehabilitation after one year if indicated, but care is required to ensure patients retain overall control of their health and well-being.

Rehabilitation is an essential part of stroke recovery for the majority of patients and should be offered to everyone requiring rehabilitation, regardless of their stroke severity. It is a dynamic process that aims to promote recovery from the direct and often devastating consequences of stroke. In those cases where recovery is no longer possible, rehabilitation aims to facilitate adjustment and ensure that individuals lead as full and meaningful a life as possible.

Interventions provided by the multi-disciplinary team aim to reduce impairments caused by stroke, promote recovery in daily life activities and ensure participation in the wider community context, for example returning to work and engaging in leisure pursuits and hobbies. Psychosocial recovery is as important, if not more so, than the physical consequences of stroke. Each team member has a valuable part to play in this process and the synergistic involvement of all rehabilitation staff is crucial in determining the potential recovery of each patient. Consequently, regular training of staff and taking part in educational sessions are fundamental parts of all stroke care provision.

When should rehabilitation start and who should be involved?

Rehabilitation should start as early as possible and not be an 'afterthought' when all acute medical interventions have been completed. Ideally, stroke rehabilitation should start on day one in an acute Stroke Unit where there is a multi-disciplinary stroke team who work together using the same philosophy of care. The core multi-disciplinary stroke team includes:

- nurse
- doctor
- occupational therapist
- physiotherapist
- speech and language therapist

Other important members of a comprehensive stroke team may include:

- psychologist
- rehabilitation assistant
- social worker
- orthotist
- orthoptist
- dietician

The benefits of stroke units are now widely accepted, with robust data confirming that patients are more likely to be alive, independent and not requiring institutional care than patients treated on general medical wards. The most recent National Sentinel Stroke Organisational Audit (RCP 2010) reported that of the 201 sites taking part, only three hospitals did not have a dedicated stroke unit.

Rehabilitation process

The rehabilitation team includes a wide variety of specialists, each of whom has their own area of expertise but also the ability to overlap their skills to ensure that the patient receives the most comprehensive and consistent care possible. The first step in the rehabilitation process is a comprehensive assessment, which is conducted by each team member. This will provide an accurate description of the patient's abilities, areas of deficit and potential for further rehabilitation input. It is crucial that the findings from these assessments are communicated to all team members, usually at weekly team meetings with relevant information inserted into clinical notes, and are not an isolated activity. Continuous assessment is necessary as the patient makes their own natural recovery from stroke, thereby ensuring that interventions are as timely and appropriate as possible.

ABC of Stroke. Edited by Jonathan Mant and Marion F Walker.
© 2011 Blackwell Publishing Ltd.

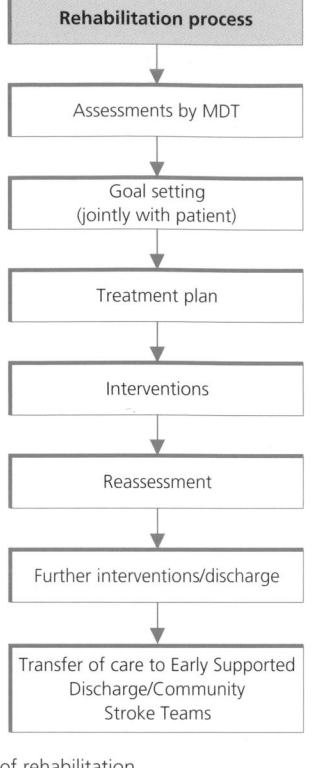

Figure 6.1 Process of rehabilitation.

To be clinically meaningful, assessments should be standardised and have proven psychometric properties. The length of time taken to administer a chosen assessment should also be considered, as lengthy assessments will prove difficult to implement in busy clinical settings. Rehabilitation goals are set between team members, in collaboration with the patient and their carer, and should be relevant to the patient's lifestyle and likely environmental discharge destination. Figure 6.1 illustrates the process of rehabilitation.

Occupational therapist

The occupational therapist is primarily concerned with promoting activities of daily living. Basic self-care tasks are always targeted first and include items such as those illustrated in Box 6.1 and Figure 6.2.

> **Box 6.1 Self-care items as assessed by the Barthel Index**
>
> Grooming
> Washing
> Dressing
> Feeding
> Toilet use
> Transferring from bed to chair
> Mobility
> Bathing
> Stairs

In addition to these self-care skills, the occupational therapist may address more instrumental tasks such as preparing food,

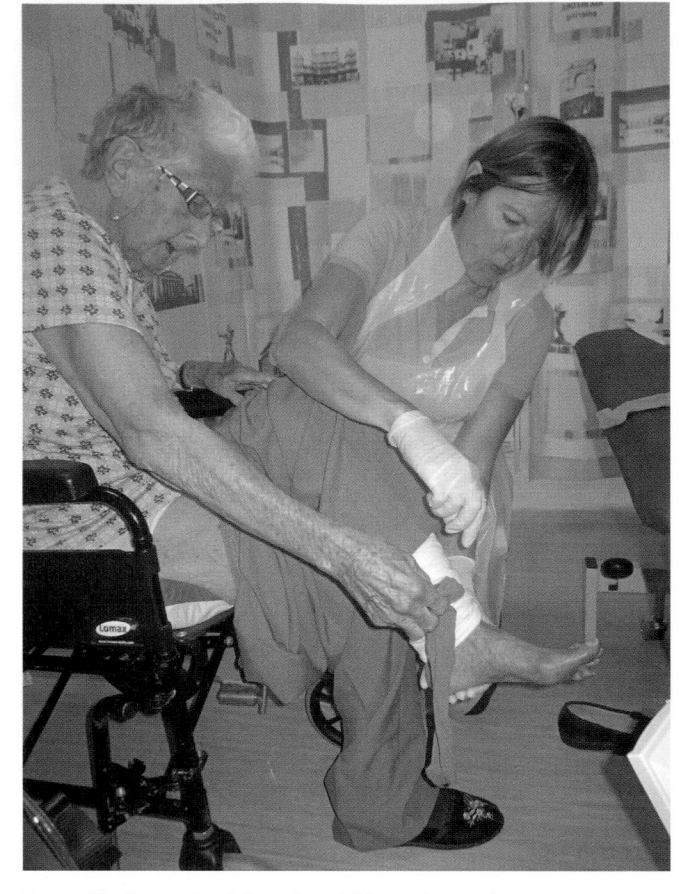

Figure 6.2 Occupational therapist teaching patient to dress.

outdoor mobility and housework, depending on the requirements of the patient and their lifestyle.

During the assessment process the occupational therapist will ascertain the nature of the patient's problem in each activity and provide specific interventions, advice or equipment that will ensure the patient reaches their optimal functional capacity. Frequently a home visit will be arranged prior to transfer of care into the community setting, to ensure that the patient is safe and that they can negotiate all environmental obstacles such as access to the property, interior stairs and safely get on and off the toilet and in and out of bed (see Figure 6.3). The home visit will indicate the environmental adaptations or aids to independence required before hospital discharge. Second stair rails, grab handles for property access and bathing equipment are commonly prescribed. The home visit also acts as a confidence-building exercise for both the patient and carer, and should reassure all parties, including health-care staff, that a return home will be successful.

The occupational therapist is also concerned with the patient's emotional and cognitive well-being. In the absence of a clinical psychology service, of which there is scarce provision in the UK, the occupational therapist may assess whether the patient has problems with mood or perceptual difficulties such as neglect or apraxia. Problems such as these have been shown to adversely affect rehabilitation progress.

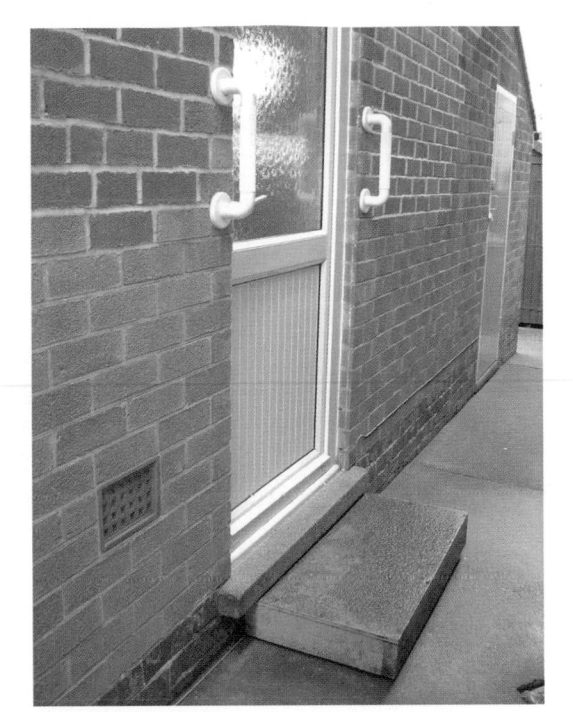

Figure 6.3 Access to house.

Physiotherapist

The physiotherapist represents the core discipline, assessing and orchestrating the patient's motor recovery following stroke. Again, a full and thorough assessment is required to assess the problematic components of all motor skills for the patient. In assessing the patient the physiotherapist will pay particular attention to:

- posture while sitting in chair/bed and while moving
- balance
- sensorimotor abilities
- strength training
- mobility
- mobility aids

The physiotherapist will ensure that the patient is comfortably positioned in bed or in a chair and is not lying or sitting in a manner that would cause harm or inhibit motor recovery. Several decades ago stroke patients were frequently assigned to bed in the early stages of recovery after stroke. We now know this to be detrimental and a contributory factor in the cause of complications such as limb oedema and deep vein thrombosis. Many stroke units encourage mobilisation on day one following stroke. Indeed, a large multi-centre randomised controlled trial is currently in progress to determine the functional implications of early mobilisation and published data to date suggest that such mobilisation (even passive movement) is not detrimental to the patient's health.

As the patient makes progress, the physiotherapist's attention will turn to standing and walking. It is obvious that in order to move, the patient will need to have sufficient balance to remain upright. Interventions may be targeted initially at getting the patient to stand with assistance and then independently, and only then

will the physiotherapist gradually incorporate dynamic standing balance before encouraging any first steps. Frequently this activity is conducted in the physiotherapy gym and may require the help of more than one member of staff and several pieces of equipment, such as a standing frame or hoist. Another key concern of the physiotherapist is the patient's ability to mobilise, either on their limbs or by using manual or electronic equipment such as a wheelchair or scooter; this will be covered in Chapter 8.

Speech and language therapists

The speech and language therapist is another core member of the stroke rehabilitation team and their initial involvement with the stroke patient may be to assess the patient's ability to swallow safely. Only when this has been achieved do they turn their attention to communication and language reacquisition. This detailed area will be covered in Chapter 9.

How much rehabilitation is beneficial?

The intensity of stroke rehabilitation in the UK and abroad has been the topic of many recent research papers (see Figure 6.4). Observational studies report that the majority of stroke patients in hospital spend their time predominantly engaged in non-therapeutic activity. The evidence would suggest that this may be due to the increased documentation and paperwork required by clinical governance procedures, along with insufficient numbers of therapy staff. Increased repetition of targeted therapeutic activities (such as dressing practice or sitting to stand) has been shown to have a beneficial impact on rehabilitation outcome. Therefore the answer to how much rehabilitation is beneficial is clear and straightforward – as much as the patient can tolerate. The provision of this intensity in the NHS is, however, problematic, and allied health profession researchers are

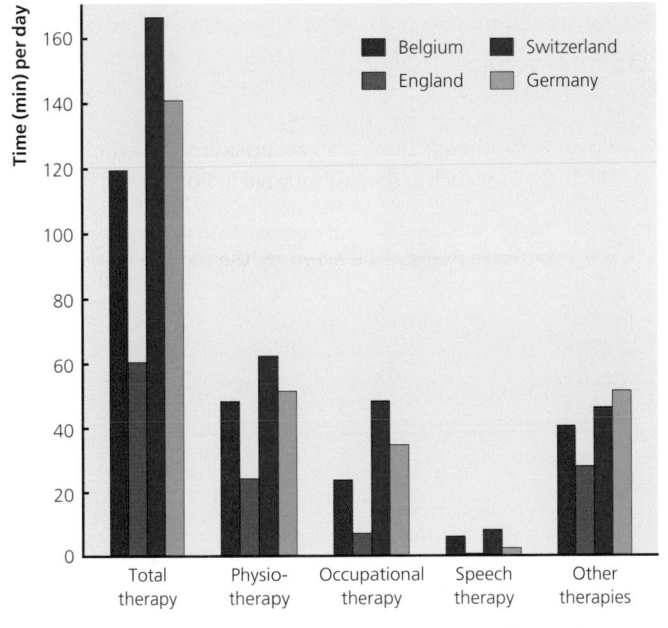

Figure 6.4 How much stroke rehabilitation across Europe (see Further reading)?

investigating ways of encouraging patient self-directed activity, for example using computer-aided and robotic technologies, especially when the patient has been transferred back into the community.

Rehabilitation following transfer of care from hospital, including Early Supported Discharge

As stated above, stroke rehabilitation ideally starts at the beginning of the patient's stay in hospital. In the UK the average length of stay following stroke is approximately three weeks. In some instances it may be desirable for patients to have their care transferred early to an Early Supported Discharge Stroke team. These teams provide a time-limited service (usually six weeks) and have been shown to facilitate equivalent levels of functional recovery to that found on stroke rehabilitation units. This service, although only appropriate for approximately 40–50% of patients with mild to moderate stroke severity, has been demonstrated to be a financially viable option to extended inpatient care and has the further advantage of patient satisfaction in returning to their chosen environment sooner. The evidence would suggest that this service should only be facilitated and conducted by a team who are skilled in the care and management of stroke patients. To date there is only limited information available on the impact of discharging patients early on the carer's level of stress.

Rehabilitation can also be provided by Community Stroke Teams, who in well-resourced areas will continue rehabilitation after discharge from the Early Supported Discharge team. In some areas rehabilitation is provided by specialist neurological outpatient clinics. Better outcomes have been found when interventions have been provided by clinicians with expertise in stroke care.

When does rehabilitation stop?

The benefits of outpatient stroke rehabilitation services have been demonstrated in a comprehensive systematic review. However, due to the limited studies available the advantages documented are restricted to the first year after stroke. Many stroke survivors will comment that they have ongoing rehabilitation needs beyond this time and that current stroke services do not have the capacity or remit to address these. The paucity of evidence to support ongoing needs is an area that urgently needs to be addressed. Further research may indicate that rehabilitation 'top-up' clinics are required or that psychosocial care interventions need to be expanded.

It is also crucial that health-care professionals ensure that the locus of control for further physical and psychological recovery, social inclusion and community participation lies with the patient, and that they do not prolong 'stroke illness' nor encourage long-term rehabilitation dependency.

Further reading

Early Supported Discharge Trialists. Services for reducing duration of hospital care for acute stroke patients. *Cochrane Database of Systematic Reviews* 2005, Issue 2.

Legg L, Langhorne P, Drummond AE, Gladman JR, Logan PA, Walker MF. Rehabilitation therapy services for stroke patients living at home: Systematic review of randomised trials. *Lancet* 2004;**363**:352–356.

Putnam K, De Wit L, Schupp W et al. A use of time by physiotherapists and occupational therapists in a stroke rehabilitation stroke unit: A comparison between four European rehabilitation centres. *Disability and Rehabilitation* 2006;**28**(22):1417–24.

RCP. *National Sentinel Stroke Audit Organisational Audit* 2010. London: Royal College of Physicians, 2010. http://www.rcplondon.ac.uk/clinical-standards/ceeu/Current-work/stroke/Documents/2010-Stroke-Public-Report.pdf.

Stroke Unit Trialists' Collaboration. Organised inpatient (stroke unit) care for stroke. *Cochrane Database of Systematic Reviews* 2007, Issue 4.

OVERVIEW

- 10% of stroke patients are of working age
- Rehabilitation services targeted at the needs of young stroke survivors are scarce
- Different Strokes is a national organisation set up by young stroke survivors to meet the needs of young stroke survivors
- A plan for a return to work after stroke should be incorporated into a rehabilitation programme early after stroke
- The sexual relationship needs of stroke patients and their carers should routinely be addressed

Often viewed as a condition of the elderly, it is less well recognised that 25% of stroke survivors are under the age of 65. Prevalence figures suggest that 10 000 individuals are under the age of 55 years and 500 children aged 15 years or less are also affected. It can be argued that the consequences of stroke are particularly devastating for those who are in the early stages of life (Box 7.1).Those of working age may have a family to support, with young children or students at university to provide for. Adults of working age may have additional responsibilities such as caring for elderly parents, who may also have significant health problems. For many stroke survivors, education may still be ongoing, with further career development a realistic option.

Box 7.1 **Example of issues affecting younger stroke patients include:**

- Loss of family role – mother, father, daughter, son
- Loss of work role
- Loss of social role – leisure and friendships
- Loss of salary or reduced income
- Loss of self-confidence
- Difficulties in caring for elderly parents
- Difficulties in sexual relationships
- Difficulties in continued education

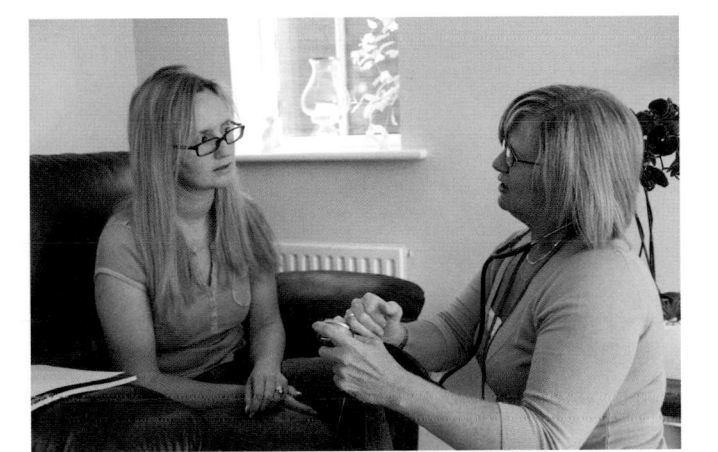

Figure 7.1 Young stroke.

Different Strokes

There are very few services that provide tailored interventions or adequately address the needs of a younger stroke population. This paucity in support and care has been voiced by young stroke survivors for many years and has resulted in the formation of a national organisation, named 'Different Strokes', which was founded in 1996. Different Strokes is a registered charity and is so called because the organisation is of the opinion that strokes in a younger age group are 'different' to those of the elderly population. It is an organisation that has been developed by young stroke survivors for young stroke survivors.

Services and support offered by Different Strokes include:

- National network of weekly exercise classes
- Website with interactive notice board (www.differentstrokes. co.uk)
- Provision of practical information
- Provision of a newsletter
- StrokeLine telephone service (0845 130 7172)
- National political voice for young stroke survivors

The issue of long-term care and the need for ongoing rehabilitation are areas of particular concern for Different Strokes and will be addressed in Chapter 12. In response to the lack of opportunity for continued physiotherapy to maintain and promote further physical

ABC of Stroke. Edited by Jonathan Mant and Marion F Walker.
© 2011 Blackwell Publishing Ltd.

recovery, Different Strokes has established a network of exercise classes. There are now 45 weekly classes across the UK and Northern Ireland and many classes are led by young stroke survivors, who have undergone professional training to become physical instructors themselves. New classes continue to be developed all the time. The organisation's website provides information on the regions involved in this service provision.

An interactive notice board is also available on the charity's website where individuals and their families can post questions to others visitors to the site. This peer support is of great psychological benefit, as stories recount successful recovery and how practical stroke problems have been tackled. For those individuals who do not have access to computers or have stroke difficulties that prevent them from accessing information in this format, a Stroke Line telephone service is available that enables stroke survivors to speak to other fellow stroke survivors, with Different Strokes acting as an intermediary for a 'stroke dateline' service. This peer support is greatly valued by those who use the service.

The lack of practical information given to stroke patients during their contact with the NHS and social care is a consistent issue highlighted by many national documents and patient involvement groups. In tackling this issue Different Strokes has developed an information pack that covers areas that are not routinely addressed by health-care services, such as sex after stroke, how to access benefits and how to return to work following stroke. So successful are these packs that approximately 50 are distributed each week across the UK. Topical information is also distributed to members via a quarterly newsletter.

Another important role of Different Strokes is to act as a national voice to raise awareness of the plight of the younger individual who has suffered a stroke. The organisation contributes to national stroke consultations such as the National Stroke Strategy (2007) and works as a key stakeholder on many political initiatives.

Return to work

The opportunity to work in paid employment is an important part of a fulfilling life. The benefits of being able to work are multiple, frequently complex and often very personal, but at the very least someone's job may define who they are, their social standing in life, and provide them with the financial means to purchase the basic comforts of life. It is therefore not difficult to understand why a return to work following stroke is a primary goal for many patients.

Every year 110 000 people in England alone suffer a stroke and more than 10% are of working age. The economic impact in terms of lost productivity and personal income is evident. The numbers of individuals returning to work following stroke varies widely and reflects the different definitions used of 'return to work'. Studies to date suggest that between 24% and 38% of patients have a successful return to work. Stroke survivors consume an estimated £689 million in benefits each year, yet health-care professionals know that many stroke survivors are relatively independent and would like to return to work.

However, even without the additional widely acknowledged complications of stroke, being without work can also have some major health implications. It can cause a loss of fitness, mental and physical deterioration, mood may be affected, patterns established through work may be disrupted, such as cycling to and from work, and there may be a loss of contact with peers and the obvious loss of income. It is crucial that health-care professionals do not under-estimate just how important a return to work is for a patient and their family, and also that they understand the psychological importance of returning to voluntary unpaid employment. It is therefore surprising that this is an area that is so frequently neglected in the care and rehabilitation of stroke patients.

Successful re-employment is influenced by intrinsic factors such as personality traits, the patient's and relatives' belief system on whether it is good to return to work regardless of recovery, and whether work will cause further damage or 'strain' on the brain. There may also be the fear of what others may think of them, especially if they work in the public sector. Extrinsic factors also play an important part in return to successful employment, such as living in an area of high unemployment, difficulty in accessing public transport and structural limitations such as limited access to buildings and the physical demands that the job entails (see Frank and Thurgood, 2006).

Vocational rehabilitation

To date, little is known about the success of vocational rehabilitation interventions for people with stroke. Most published research has addressed people with traumatic brain injury or incorporated those with a diagnosis of brain injury, including those with stroke, TBI and other causes, thereby obscuring what may be important differences in rehabilitation needs. For people with traumatic brain injury there is evidence to suggest that specialist vocational rehabilitation programmes are successful (50–70% in work) and cost effective, with costs recovered in around 20 months and long-term benefits over seven years or more. However, evidence for people with stroke is lacking at present. The majority of vocational rehabilitation interventions are delivered by community or hospital-based outreach teams, for which there is little supporting research evidence. It is unclear what happens to people who do not have access to these services, how those from ethnic minority groups are affected or how helpful interventions targeting them may be.

Anecdotal evidence suggests that vocational rehabilitation interventions need to be targeted early after stroke, with the occupational therapist making contact with the employer very soon after the onset of stroke. This early contact ensures that an avenue for further discussion is open when the severity and resultant deficits from stroke are clear. Ensuring that good communication links remain between employer and employee facilitates an understanding of the problems caused by stroke and how the therapist, patient and employer can work together to ensure a successful return to work. Over the course of the initial stroke recovery, regular discussions can take place as to the best methods of returning to the same job or, if this is not possible, what alternative jobs may be appropriate.

Ongoing support is also required when a return to work has taken place, as retention in employment is a known problematic area for many stroke patients. For those who wish to return to work and are unable to do so, help and counselling may be required to adjust to a work-free life and to identify alternative ways to channel productive energy.

Sex after stroke

The ability to have an intimate relationship with our partner is highly valued in health and should be no less so following a stroke. Sadly, discussion of this topic causes great discomfort and embarrassment and is very rarely addressed by health-care staff or broached by patients themselves. Due to hospitalisation, many individuals may give this topic little thought and may only consider the implications for their relationship some time after discharge from hospital. There are many reasons that may cause a reduced intimacy between partners following stroke and some are listed in Box 7.2.

Box 7.2 **Reasons for reduced sexual activity**

- Excessive tiredness
- Failure to sustain a comfortable position
- Side effects from medication (e.g. impotence)
- Loss of self-esteem, self-image and confidence
- Loss of libido in partner (e.g. carer strain, fear of causing harm)
- Pain
- Limb weakness
- Sensory loss
- Fear of raising blood pressure and causing another stroke
- Depression
- Anxiety

It may be that the individual who has sustained the stroke feels less attractive and a burden, especially if the partner has to attend to their personal care needs and hygiene. The partner may also be over-protective and not wish to make demands of a sexual nature for fear of delaying stroke recovery. It is therefore vital that couples are open about their fears and explore their concerns about resuming their sex life with each other if any progress is to be made. Where language is a problem following stroke, the speech and language therapist can assist in helping the individual to develop effective ways of communicating their thoughts and fears to their partner.

The role of the general practitioner is also very important in addressing intimacy issues when the patient has settled back into their home environment. The effects of drugs can be discussed and alternatives tried if it is felt that the present drug regime is causing a loss of libido. Alternative sexual positions and an exchange of dominant partner can be suggested to ensure that the individual is comfortable and is experiencing no pain. Reassurance that full sexual intercourse is not the only way to achieve intimacy may relieve the pressure of sexual performance in the early stages of returning home. Referral to self-help leaflets provided by the Stroke Association (www.stroke.org.uk) may be helpful, or a counsellor may be required when emotional and relationship communications do not seem to be resolving.

Further reading

Frank, AO, Thurgood, J. Vocational rehabilitation in the UK: Opportunities for the health care professions. *International Journal of Therapy and Rehabilitation* 2006;**13**:126–34.

McCrum R. *My Year Off: Rediscovering life after a stroke*. Portland, OR: Broadway Books, 1998.

Radford K, Walker MF. Impact of stroke on return to work. *Brain Impairment* 2008;**9**(2):161–9.

CHAPTER 8

Mobility

Marion F Walker

University of Nottingham, Nottingham, UK

OVERVIEW

- Approximately 80% of stroke survivors resume walking in the first year after stroke
- Perceptual and cognitive problems may limit mobility independence
- Mobility aids are commonly prescribed, but regular review is required to ensure correct usage
- Where possible, carers should be involved in mobility rehabilitation
- Orthoses may be required to assist mobility after stroke
- A return to driving after stroke should occur after appropriate assessment by relevant health-care professionals and, if appropriate, a regional driving centre

An inability to mobilise independently following stroke is common and the desire to remedy this is frequently at the top of stroke survivors' immediate wish list. Bed mobility will be assessed by the physiotherapist very early after stroke and the patient will be taught how best to position themselves and how to relieve body pressure by turning in bed. The ability to transfer safely is a crucial step in returning to full mobility and this will involve a transfer from bed to chair, on and off the toilet and from a chair to a standing position. Fortunately, approximately 80% of patients in the first year after stroke will resume walking.

Muscle weakness and increased tone may not be the only factors prohibiting mobility performance, and sensory, ataxia and perceptual problems should also be considered as limitations with an impact on independence. A flaccid lower limb is a common initial presentation, with tone increasing over days and weeks. A typical stroke gait is one of a flexed hip, leg internally rotated and adducted, extended knee, with the foot inverted and in plantar flexion.

Walking after a stroke with the increased possibility of a subsequent fall is anxiety provoking for many individuals, therefore a thorough assessment by the physiotherapist and a gradual return to mobility are necessary, with standing balance independence a prerequisite. The physiotherapist will instruct the patient and their carer on the safest methods of getting off the floor if a fall has

occurred. This will increase the patient and carer's confidence to cope on returning home should a fall occur. Indeed, it is essential that carers are fully involved in all aspects of the patient's mobility recovery.

'Stepping' is usually the first stage of a return to walking and this is practised in environments such as the physiotherapy gym, with one or two additional assistants present so that the patient feels supported and safe. For those who require more physical support, a standing frame may be required to increase standing balance before stepping is attempted.

Quality of gait

The quality of walking gait is a priority in physiotherapy practice and much time and effort is spent on improving this. While this is an admirable goal to strive for, it is actually very difficult without sophisticated measurement analysis equipment to measure in an objective way. Attempts to evaluate walking gait among physiotherapists have demonstrated that it is a very unreliable measure of stroke recovery. There are, however, other measures that provide robust meaningful data, such as the '10-metre timed walking test'. This measure has been shown to be simple to carry out, requires no equipment, and is a valid, reliable and sensitive measure of walking recovery.

Walking aids

Ideally, a stroke patient will return to independent walking, but in some cases walking aids are required and may become a permanent fixture in daily life following stroke. Varieties of walking aids are available and are usually administered following a detailed assessment by the physiotherapist. Walking frames and rollators that increase the patient's stability while moving are sometimes used for continued balance problems. Walking sticks are the most common mobility devices supplied.

Regular checks should be made to ensure the safety of all mobility equipment provided, such as the renewal of worn rubber ferrules, and to confirm that the equipment is still being used in the correct way originally demonstrated. As with all rehabilitation activities, the health-care professional should ensure that all patients are using prescribed visual and hearing aids and that these are in good

---

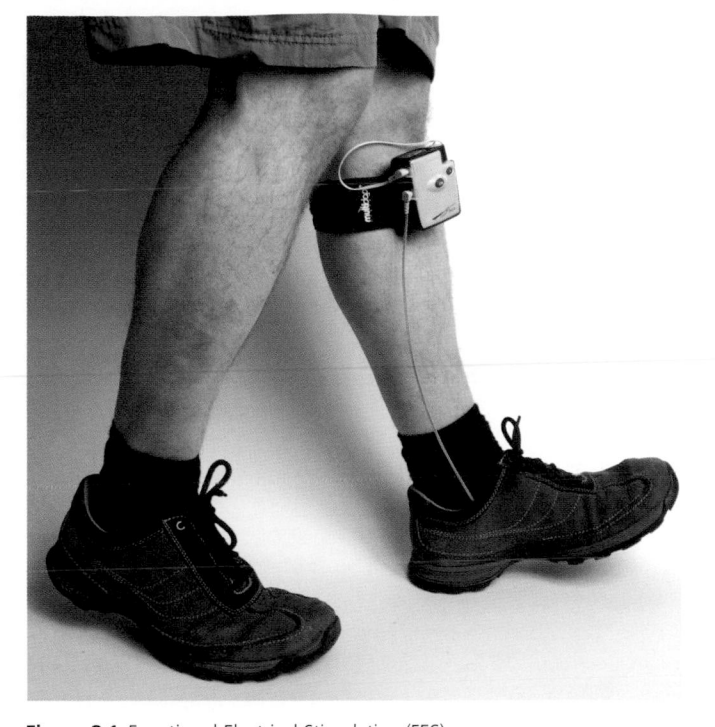

Figure 8.1 Functional Electrical Stimulation (FES).

and working condition. Such aids are particularly important if the patient is mobilising outside.

For some patients an additional facilitatory aid may be required to assist mobility such as an external ankle foot orthosis, which controls the position and motion of the ankle and can also be designed to have an indirect impact on the knee joint. Functional Electrical Stimulation (FES) can be applied by skin surface electrodes or implanted electrodes, producing contractions in the ankle muscles by means of electrical stimulation (Figure 8.1). Ankle foot orthoses and FES are commonly used to compensate for foot drop after stroke.

Environmental considerations

Appropriate footwear should be discussed with the patient and their family on admission to the stroke rehabilitation ward. The occupational therapist or physiotherapist will provide advice on the most suitable forms. Most patients feel comfortable in training shoes or flat, supportive shoes that give additional ankle support. Similarly, appropriate comfortable clothing will be advised, such as jogging trousers that ensure the patient has maximum movement while exercising.

During a hospital stay walking is made less problematic by practising on uncarpeted surfaces. The foot can easily glide on the smooth surface with little resistance. The importance of walking on different surfaces should therefore be acknowledged to ensure that the patient has confidence walking over all terrains, such as carpeted areas, grass, uneven ground and pavements with differing heights of kerb.

During the pre-discharge home visit (already discussed in Chapter 6) advice will be given on the importance of keeping floor spaces free from clutter such as hearth rugs and carpet runners.

Advice to keep pets in another room while the patient adjusts to their home environment will also ensure walking safety and help prevent falls.

Further mobility guidance and assistance provided by the physiotherapist may need to continue after transfer of care from hospital and can be provided in outpatient clinics or as part of community stroke teams. A re-referral to physiotherapy for mobility problems may be worth considering after stroke, as functional recovery can continue long after the completion of motor recovery.

Wheelchair provision

Many physiotherapists may not wish to consider the use of a wheelchair early after stroke, instead focusing on improving balance and independent mobility. However, in cases of severe stroke the provision of a wheelchair may be indicated. The psychological impact of wheelchair provision should also be considered, as it may be viewed by the patient as giving up on the possibility of walking again. Careful discussion with the patient and their carer should highlight the reasons for such wheelchair use, especially as mobility recovery has been documented to occur over lengthy periods. The physiotherapist may feel that a wheelchair is only required for long distances outside, thereby ensuring that the patient fully integrates back into society.

For some patients, the only mobility available may be through the provision of a permanent wheelchair. In such cases, extra comfort such as sheepskin blankets and pressure-relief seating is an essential part of the wheelchair assessment.

Manual wheelchairs are commonly supplied to stroke patients and can be ordered after a full assessment from wheelchair services with left- or right-side steering propulsion. In elderly patients or those who wish to undertake longer distances, carer-propelled or electric wheelchairs may also be ordered. The patient and their family need to be instructed on the general care of such equipment and regular checks for battery life. Patients with perceptual or cognitive difficulties may be unable to operate wheelchairs for obvious reasons of safety.

Independent advice and guidance on mobility issues can be obtained from the charity Ricability, www.ricability.org.uk.

Driving

All drivers are required to notify the DVLA (Driver and Vehicle Licensing Agency) of their stroke or transient ischaemic attack and are automatically precluded from driving for a period of one month, regardless of stroke severity. Health-care professionals should ensure that all patients who drive have access to this information. If after a period of one month the patient's general practitioner considers them fit to drive, they may do so. If the doctor advises against returning to driving, it is the patient's responsibility to notify the DVLA of this decision and also to notify their car insurance company. However, it should be acknowledged that many general practitioners do not have sufficient time or adequate training to detect other non-physical components of return to driving, such as lack of concentration or subtle cognitive

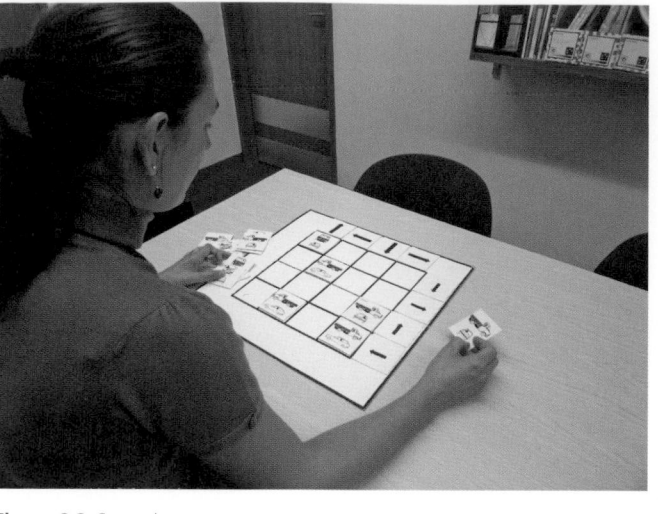

Figure 8.2 Screening assessment.

impairments, and that it is advisable to request further help in making the decision whether to return to driving or not.

A simple screening assessment called the Nottingham Stroke Drivers Screening Assessment can be conducted by an occupational therapist, which will indicate cognitive and perceptual competence to drive (Figure 8.2). This test takes approximately 30 minutes to administer and has proven specificity and sensitivity. If the patient passes this, they are then recommended to undertake further testing, including an on-the-road test, at a regional driving centre to ensure road safety and to be assessed and advised on any physical adaptations required to their vehicle.

Physical impairments can be overcome by making adaptations to the car, such as assisted steering wheel knobs so that the car may be driven with one hand (Figure 8.3). Foot pedals can also be relocated to unconventional positions.

The Blue Badge Scheme is a national scheme that allows preferential parking for those with a disability affecting mobility. Individuals with restrictive mobility problems can also access this scheme if

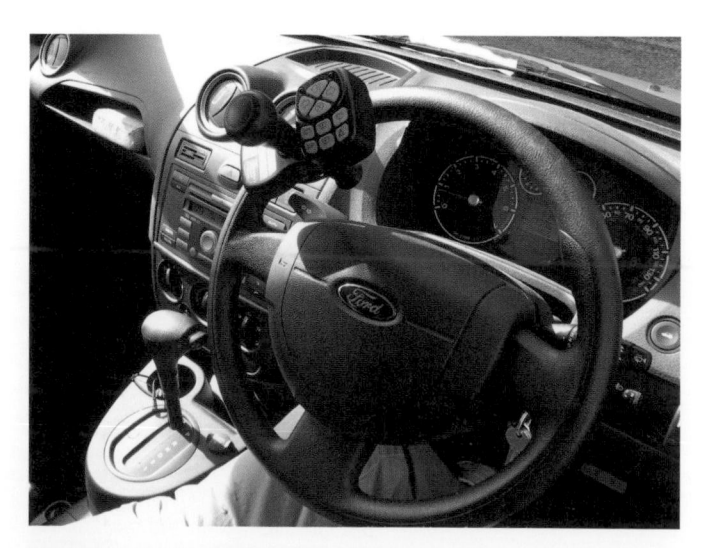

Figure 8.3 Steering wheel.

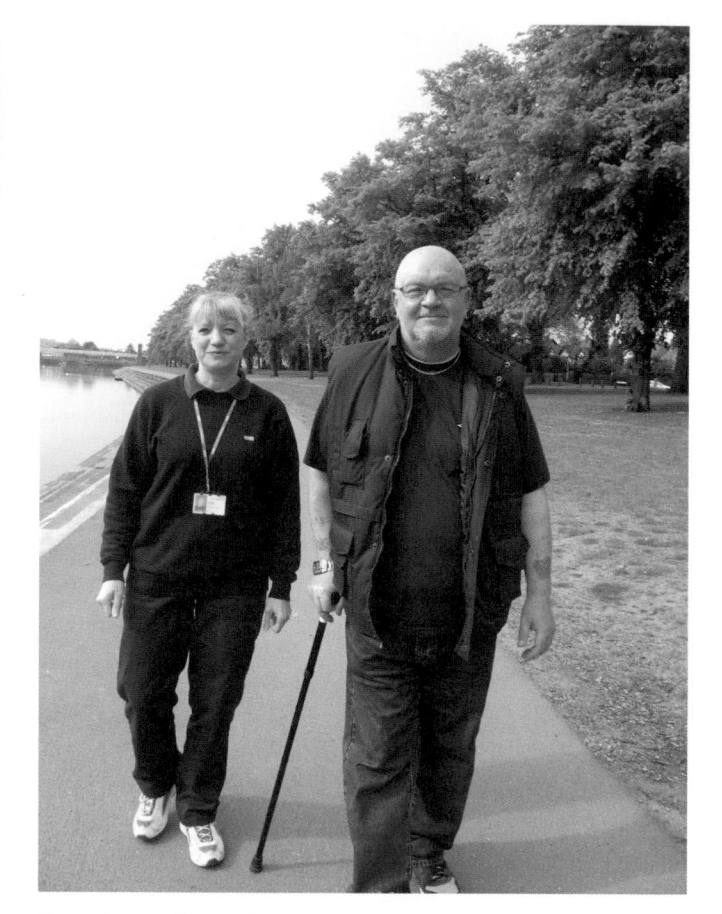

Figure 8.4 Outdoor mobility.

they are passengers in vehicles owned by other family members or carers. Further information on eligibility for this scheme can be accessed via the patient's local council or through the Department of Transport.

Adjuncts to mobility retraining

Several small studies have investigated the value of assistive devices to physiotherapy mobility practice. Treadmill training with some body weight supported in an overhead harness has been used by some physiotherapists to re-educate in walking. However, the evidence to date is not sufficiently robust to recommend that this become an integral part of routine clinical care. The cost of such equipment and the necessary space required to house such a device are also prohibitive in most physiotherapy departments.

Outdoor mobility

A large proportion of patients do not resume outdoor mobility even when they are physically capable of doing so. Recent research studies have reported that 42% of stroke patients do not get out of the house as often as they would like, citing a fear of falling, lack of confidence and lack of information as the main reasons for this restriction. Mobility programmes exist in other countries such as America and Australia, but to date no such dedicated service exists in the UK (Figure 8.4).

There has been some suggestion that such an outdoor mobility programme is likely to be bebeficial. From research conducted in one centre in England a mean of 7 visits were administered over a period of 16 weeks. Interventions such as practising getting on and off buses, walking outside over uneven ground, and intensive practice with electric scooters, travelling in taxis and so on were commonplace. The researchers found that stroke patients receiving such visits were more likely to get out of the house as often as they wanted and that they undertook more than double the number of journeys outside than patients who did not receive this service. This intervention is currently part of a national multi-centre randomised controlled study in the UK to confirm if the results from the single-centre study are generalisable to the general population.

Further reading

Lincoln NB, Fanthome Y. Reliability of the Stroke Drivers Screen Assessment. *Clinical Rehabilitation* 1994;**8**:157–60.

Logan P, Gladman JRF, Avery A, Walker MF, Dyas J, Groom L. Randomised controlled trial of an occupational therapy intervention to increase outdoor mobility after stroke. *British Medical Journal* 2004;**329**:1372.

Weerdesteyn V, de Niet M, van Duijnhoven HJ, Geurts AC. Falls in individuals with stroke. *Journal of Rehabilitation Research and Development* 2008;**45**(8):1195–213.

CHAPTER 9

Communication and Swallowing

Pam Enderby

School of Health and Related Research, University of Sheffield, Sheffield, UK

OVERVIEW

- All patients with speech and language or other communication problems should be assessed by a speech and language therapist to determine the nature of the difficulty and rehabilitation potential
- Comprehension and perseveration should be taken into account when determining mental capacity
- Difficulties with speech, language and communication have a significant effect on the well-being and mood of the patient and the family
- There is research evidence to support the contribution of specific speech and language therapy techniques to improving communication outcomes
- While the most significant recovery from speech, language and communication deficits takes place in the first three to six months, many patients continue to improve over several years
- All stroke patients should be screened to identify the presence of swallowing disorders at the earliest opportunity
- Identifying dysphagia and instigating appropriate management reduces mortality and morbidity
- Speech and language therapists play a key role in the assessment and management of swallowing disorders

The most important issue in the care of a person who has suffered a stroke is correctly identifying the associated symptoms in order that appropriate management can be instigated immediately. There is strong evidence that diagnosing the nature and severity of any speech, language, cognitive or swallowing deficit has an impact on the progress and final outcome of the patient, as well as improving team management and helping patients and relatives in coping with the sequelae.

Aphasia

Identifying the nature and type of these problems is not as easy as one would first think. General ill-health, confusion and shock can mask or be mistaken for aphasia.

Aphasia is defined as a defect or loss of the power of expression through language which includes writing and gesture (see Box 9.1). It has an impact on the ability to comprehend both spoken and written language. This definition rightly infers a spectrum of disorders of both expression and comprehension that are attributable to cerebral dysfunction.

Box 9.1 Definitions

Aphasia is a language disorder
Dysarthria is a speech disorder
Dyspraxia is a motor programming disorder

In general, dysphasia is associated with a lesion in the dominant hemisphere, with non-fluent dysphasia being more likely to be due to a lesion of the dominant frontal lobe and fluent aphasia to be due to more posterior lesions. Typically, most patients with stroke have a combination, referred to as a mixed or global aphasia, and this occurs with extensive lesions within the middle cerebral artery territory. A fluent aphasia is apparent when the person speaks fluently, using good intonation, but does not make any sense and frequently speaks with nonsense words. This aphasia is often associated with severe comprehension problems.

It is important to look out for:

- *Perseveration* – when an individual repeats a word inappropriately. For example, an individual may repeat the word 'yes' when they mean 'no'.
- *Confabulation* – when an individual fills in the gaps in conversation by making up stories to cover their word-finding difficulty.

The prefix 'dys' used to be employed to infer a lesser degree of severity of the problem, whereas the prefix 'a' indicated a total loss. However, today these terms are used interchangeably and thus the terms aphasia, anarthria and apraxia are not employed to indicate any difference in severity to the terms dysphasia, dysarthria and dyspraxia.

How many people are dysphasic?

Of the 220 persons per 100 000 population who have a first or recurrent stroke, each year 65 will become dysphasic. Of these,

ABC of Stroke. Edited by Jonathan Mant and Marion F Walker.
© 2011 Blackwell Publishing Ltd.

it is suggested that approximately one third will recover their language skills fully. The severity of the dysphasia at seven days after the stroke has been found to be a good predictor of eventual recovery. However, approximately 10% of patients will recover more language function than predicted and 10% will do less well. It has been suggested that previous cognitive function, age, the site and size of the lesion, as well as personality, literacy levels, educational attainment and social circumstances, in addition to speech and language therapy and rehabilitation, can influence recovery.

Impact of aphasia

The social impact of dysphasia cannot be under-estimated. The inability to express oneself, one's concerns, personality and humour, can erode self-image and confidence rapidly. In addition, it is hard to truly appreciate the fear, anger and frustration when the inability to speak is compounded by difficulties in understanding not only what people are saying but also anything that is written. Thus it is not surprising that people with aphasia are frequently found to be clinically depressed.

Screening tests and intervention

There are several different tests that can be conducted by any health-care professional to indicate specific language disorders. It is particularly important to establish the patient's level of comprehension in order to ensure that consent to treatment and engagement in rehabilitation are appropriately managed.

One such screening test is the Frenchay Aphasia Screening Test, which has been found to be simple to use and has good psychometric properties. More in-depth and detailed assessment will be carried out by the speech and language therapist, who can provide information on deficits as well as retained abilities that can assist the rehabilitation team and family in improving the effectiveness of communication with the patient. These detailed assessments are required in order to determine the speech and language therapy schedule. Targeted speech and language therapy has been found to be efficacious for certain people with dysphasia. In addition, appropriate attention, general stimulation and support are appreciated by patients and relatives and have an impact on social recovery.

Dysarthria

Dysarthria is a motor speech disorder affecting the ability to articulate and phonate, rendering speech less intelligible. People with dysarthria alone will be able to read, write and gesture, which discriminates them from those with dysphasia. Dysarthria following stroke is usually associated with bilateral hemisphere damage or can occur with a stroke affecting the cerebellum, which is likely to result in the speech being over-loud and poorly coordinated. A high proportion of people with dysarthria following a stroke will show rapid recovery within the first seven days. Any residual dysarthria may recover slowly over many months.

Dyspraxia

Dyspraxia is a difficulty in performing complex tasks consciously because of a lack of purposeful motor control. It causes a difficulty in performing complex tasks consciously, while unconscious or automatic tasks may remain intact. Thus an individual may have no difficulty in licking their lips but would have difficulty in sticking out their tongue on command. They may be able to speak clearly for automatic utterances, such as saying the days of the week, but not be able to say something specific.

Speech and language therapy

Speech and language therapy aims to reduce the impairment of the speech and language problem with targeted specific speech and language exercises, to assist the individual in communicating as effectively as possible (this may be through speech or a technical device) and to help participation in social activities by improving confidence and developing strategies.

Box 9.2 gives golden rules for talking to someone with a speech or language problem following a stroke.

Box 9.2 Golden rules for talking to someone with a speech and language problem following a stroke

- Speak more slowly than is usual – but avoid being patronising
- Reduce distractions in the room – turn off the television
- Check frequently that the person is understanding you
- Repeat what you say but use different language – phrase it differently
- Make sure that you listen to their attempts to speak – pick up intonation and facial expression
- Do not speak more loudly than is appropriate – but check if they are wearing their hearing aid
- Use your facial expression and intonation to convey additional meaning
- Do not pretend to understand if you do not
- Encourage the person to point, draw or use gestures
- Keep relaxed!

Swallowing problems

Between 30% and 40% of conscious stroke clients have significant dysphagia on the day of the stroke and 15% to 20% at one week poststroke. At one month poststroke 2% of stroke survivors will have swallowing problems.

Normal swallowing requires the interaction of many systems and muscle groups and thus it is not surprising that it can be disrupted by a stroke. Usually food is placed within the mouth, the lips close, and the tongue moves the food around the mouth and between the teeth for chewing. This is called the oral phase. Following this the bollus is collected by a guttering of the tongue, the soft palate raises and the bollus is propelled into the pharynx, where the larynx has lifted to form a seal against the epiglottis. This is called the pharyngeal phase (see Figure 9.1).

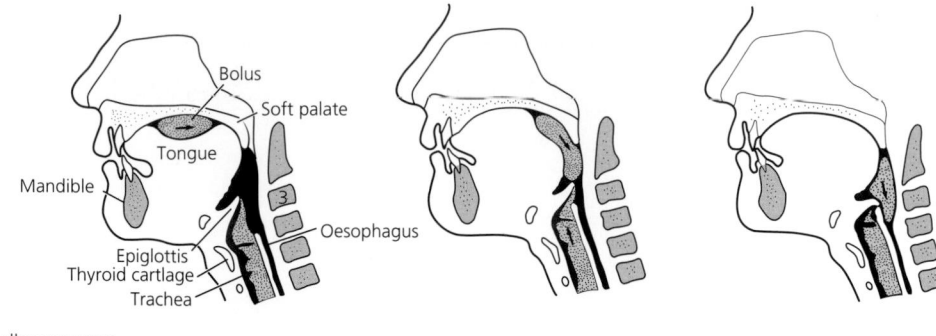

Figure 9.1 Normal swallow process.

Detecting a problem with swallowing is essential, as it can have a direct impact on the patient's outcome. Danger signals are indicated in Box 9.3. It is also important to note that an effective gag reflex does not indicate that the individual can swallow effectively.

Box 9.3 **Danger signals of swallowing problems**

- The voice sounds wet or husky
- The person has a weak, ineffective cough
- The person coughs frequently when eating or drinking
- The person has dysarthria
- Food and drink leak out of the mouth
- The person does not sit upright when eating
- The person is semi-conscious
- Food is retained in the mouth

The speech and language therapist will undertake a detailed swallowing assessment if there is any indication of a problem in this area. In some cases a short period of 'nil by mouth' and alternative hydration and nutrition is required, whereas with others an adapted diet (softened or thickened) may be warranted. Additional security can be afforded by attending to the feeding position, the size of the mouthful and the position of the head while eating.

Further reading

Byng S, Jones E. Therapy for the language impairment in aphasia. In: (eds) Greenwood RJ, Barnes M, McMillan TM, Ward C. *Handbook of Neurological Rehabilitation*, 2nd edn. New York: Psychology Press, 2003.

Cichero J. Swallowing rehabilitation. In: (eds) Cichero J, Murdoch B. *Dysphagia Foundation, Theory and Practice*. Chichester: John Wiley and Sons, Ltd, 2006.

Enderby P. Dysarthria. In: (eds) GreenwoodRJ, Barnes M, McMillan TM, Ward C. *Handbook of Neurological Rehabilitation*, 2nd edn. New York: Psychology Press, 2003.

Enderby P, Wood V, Wade D. (2006) *Frenchay Aphasia Screening Test*, 2nd edn. Chichester: John Wiley and Sons Ltd.

CHAPTER 10

Psychological Problems after Stroke

Jane Barton

Sheffield Health and Social Care Foundation, NHS Trust, , Sheffield, UK

OVERVIEW

- For many people a stroke will be seen as a traumatic event and is likely to evoke an emotional response, ranging from a normal grieving response to more serious emotional disorders
- Depression and anxiety are the most common psychological problems following stroke, with approximately 30–40% of patients being affected by one or both of these disorders
- The presence of emotional disorders that remain untreated can have a significant negative impact on the degree and quality of recovery that a patients achieves
- It is essential that patients are routinely assessed for mood disorders, by appropriately trained staff
- Treatments and interventions should be evidence based and tailored to individual patient needs
- All members of a multi-disciplinary team have a part to play in the psychological care that is given to stroke patients

Table 10.1 Model of adjustment.

Shock
'I can't believe this has happened'
'This has come completely out of the blue'

Denial, disbelief
'I don't actually believe I have had a stroke. . . I'll be OK in a few days'
'I'd be all right if I was in my own home'

Grief, mourning and depression
'I feel so hopeless now that I cannot walk. . . my life will never be the same again'
'I used to be a lively, energetic person. . . now I feel like hibernating away from everyone'

Anger
'I wish I'd stopped smoking earlier'
'The care that you get in hospital is terrible. . . nobody bothers with you'

Adjustment
'I can't walk the distances that I used to, but I can use my car to get to the places that I need to now'
'I may not be able to talk as well as I did before, but I have found a successful way of communicating with people that I know well'

There is now increasing recognition that having a stroke can, and very often does, lead to a range of emotional experiences of varying severity. The most common mood disorders that occur are associated with either depression or anxiety, or both, and are estimated to affect around one third of all patients. It is important to recognise that not all stroke patients will develop emotional disorders, but that the majority will experience significant emotional distress.

Emotional distress

Feelings of distress are very common following a stroke, and are understood to be part of a natural process of emotional and behavioural adjustment. Emotions experienced include shock, disbelief, anger and frustration. Patients often ask: 'Why has this happened to me?', 'What have I done to deserve this?' These feelings of distress have been likened to the process of grieving following a bereavement, in the case of stroke the loss of a former sense of self and lifestyle. In many cases the stroke patient is able to work through these feelings and find a way of adjusting to their new life circumstances. Table 10.1 shows the model of emotional adjustment. However, for some this remains more of a struggle, and depression may develop.

Depression and anxiety

Between 20% and 50% of stroke patients are believed to be depressed at any one time. The timing of onset is believed to vary, with some people more likely to be depressed in the early days following their stroke, while for others the depression onset may be much later. Critical times when patients appear to be particularly vulnerable to their mood worsening are first when a patient is discharged home from hospital, and the experience of being back in their own home highlights to them the extent of their disability. Patients often think that while they may have struggled to make a cup of tea with the occupational therapist when in hospital, they will be fully competent at this task if they are at home in their own kitchen, when in fact they are not. This can often be the moment of realisation for many patients, and as such can lead to a significant worsening of their mood. The second critical time is reaching the end of rehabilitation, which can often be difficult for patients. If the

ABC of Stroke. Edited by Jonathan Mant and Marion F Walker.
© 2011 Blackwell Publishing Ltd.

Table 10.2 Risk factors associated with depression.

Major risk factors and indicators
• Past history (or family history) of depression (or severe emotional distress)
• Low social support
• Associated disability
• Persistence of symptoms over two weeks
• Suicidal thoughts
• Self-neglect
• Psychotic symptoms

patient, for example, is still not able either to walk independently or communicate effectively, realising that no amount of continued therapy will lead to improvement may often develop the sinking feeling of 'this is as good as it is going to get', and a significant drop in mood may follow.

Although there is an organic basis for some depression following stroke, a number of psychosocial variables are also relevant, as the experience of depression appears to be associated with the losses that people perceive to result from the stroke. Certain risk factors are known to be associated with the development of depression. These are detailed in Table 10.2. In some more extreme cases patients may develop a pervading sense of hopelessness regarding the future, and feelings of depression can become so severe that people feel that they no longer want to continue living. It is estimated that stroke patients are at twice the risk of the general population of committing suicide, and that this risk is greater in younger people, if they have already had a previous stroke, and if they only spend a short time in hospital. In the majority of cases suicidal ideation is strongly associated with having a diagnosis of severe depression.

Anxiety following a stroke can take a number of forms. The most common are feelings of generalised anxiety, where the patient worries excessively about everything; feelings of panic, which result in episodes of hyperventilation, with the patient often misattributing this to having a further stroke; phobias about various objects or situations that the patient associates with the stroke, or avoidance of re-entering social situations; and symptoms of posttraumatic stress, often in the form of flashbacks to the actual stroke event.

Impact of emotional distress on recovery

The presence of emotional distress can often have a significant negative impact on a patient's rehabilitation and recovery, as patients will inevitably engage less well in their rehabilitation. In the case of depression, those patients whose depression remains untreated actually make fewer functional gains in the longer term. Untreated depression is also associated with a greater likelihood of patient death. This is perhaps not surprising when we think about how depression manifests, in that people who are depressed are more likely to withdraw and become avoidant, perhaps failing to participate in their therapy and rehabilitation, and may fail to take their secondary prevention medication or to eat properly, and generally take less care of themselves and their overall well-being. It is therefore fundamentally important that depression is assessed and treated correctly at all times following a stroke. The National Clinical Guidelines for Stroke, published by the Royal College

of Physicians (2008), give detailed information on the correct assessment and management of all psychological disorders that arise following stroke.

Assessment of mood disorders

Assessing depression and anxiety in stroke patients is a complicated task. The difficulty is that a stroke patient may have a range of problems, including cognitive dysfunction and speech- and language-related difficulties, which make assessment difficult, as many features of ischaemic brain injury may be misattributed to depression. Table 10.3 details some of the more common signs and symptoms of depression and anxiety. It is important, therefore, to find the most appropriate assessment tool for the particular needs of the patient. Thomas (2009) provides an overview of the different methods and assessment techniques for assessing depression in stroke patients.

Assessment of either depression or anxiety should follow the guidance published by the National Institute for Health and Clinical Excellence (2009). In this, a hierarchical system of assessment and diagnosis is advocated, whereby the initial screening of patient mood is undertaken by non-specialist mental health professionals. The screening tools have cut-off scores indicating if the person is likely to be suffering from depression or some mood-related disorder. This process in itself does not provide a diagnosis, but rather is an indication that the person may well be suffering from depression and that a thorough diagnostic interview should then be undertaken based on formal diagnostic criteria.

Treatment of emotional disorders

Knowing when and how best to intervene, and by whom the intervention is best delivered, is complex. Following the stepped model

Table 10.3 Signs and symptoms of depression and anxiety.

Depression Signs and symptoms	Anxiety Signs and symptoms
Thoughts and feelings	*Thoughts and feelings*
I can't cope	Constant worrying
I am to blame	What if this happens again?
Hopelessness	What will people think of me?
Negative outlook (self, future)	What if I can't cope?
Sadness	How will I manage at home?
Suicidal thoughts	How will I communicate with my family?
Tearfulness	
Behaviour	*Behaviour*
Social withdrawal	Avoidance
Apathy	Withdrawal
Inactivity	Increased activity
Avoidance	Ritualised behaviours
Physical	*Physical*
Poor concentration	Palpitations
Poor memory	Chest pain
Fatigue and listlessness	Butterflies in stomach
Disturbed appetite	Dry mouth
Disturbed sleep	Sweating
	Breathlessness

approach advocated by NICE, the least intrusive, most effective intervention ought to be offered first. The increasing complexity of the depression presentation is then matched by increasingly complex and specialist interventions, which are delivered by specialists trained in treating mental health problems. The key to successful management of emotional disorders in stroke patients is therefore to have an accurate assessment of the severity of the disorder, in order that the most effective treatment can be offered.

Mild to moderate depression

Many stroke patients often present with either sub-threshold depression, or depression of a mild to moderate degree. In such cases, there is a range of recommended evidence-based interventions that can often be delivered by non-mental health professionals. Table 10.4 shows some of the recommendations from NICE, adapted for use with stroke patients.

For many patients, talking through the events of the stroke can be crucial in helping the patient and the family to emotionally process the trauma of the stroke event. Individual or family counselling can be effective, as can more group-based approaches. Having the opportunity to process and reflect on what has actually happened to them and to share common experiences can be extremely beneficial. Using a framework that describes a typical approach to grieving can be extremely helpful in normalising the process of emotional adjustment for patients following their stroke.

Table 10.4 Interventions for sub-threshold and mild-moderate depression following stroke.

Sleep hygiene
Establish regular sleep and wake times
Create a proper environment for sleep
Avoid excess eating, drinking alcohol or smoking before sleep
Regular physical exercise

Active monitoring
Discuss presenting problem
Provide information about depression
Arrange follow-up assessment
Make contact if the patient does not attend appointments

Low-intensity psychosocial interventions
Physical activity programmes modified for stroke; peer support programme in a group with other stroke patients
Individual guided self-help based on CBT principles
Computerised CBT

Drug treatment
Do not use antidepressants routinely, but consider them for patients with:
- a past history of moderate or severe depression
- mild depression that complicates the care of the stroke
- initial presentation of sub-threshold depressive symptom present for at least two years
- or sub-threshold depressive symptoms or mild depression persisting after other interventions

Source: Adapted from National Institute for Health and Clinical Excellence. Depression in adults with a chronic physical health problem. *Clinical Guideline 91*. London: NICE, 2009.

Moderate to severe depression

For those stroke patients who present with a more severe depression, a range of interventions is suggested. These include high-intensity psychological interventions as well as antidepressant medication. In all cases, interventions will usually be delivered by trained specialists.

Cognitive behavioural therapy (CBT) is an extremely effective intervention for older people who are depressed. CBT approaches tend to focus on helping clients to challenge and evaluate their negative styles of thinking, and to replace these with more adaptive and realistic thinking patterns. This approach can be helpful with patients who may catastrophise the negative outcomes of their stroke. Behaviour therapy is another type of psychological therapy that is known to be helpful. The theory underpinning this is that mood is linked to behaviour, and that increasing the positive experiences that people have will lead to an improvement in mood. With stroke patients, building previously enjoyed activities and interests into the day can be extremely helpful and have a positive impact on mood. However, most patients who are depressed find it extremely difficult to motivate themselves to engage in activities, which is why professional involvement is crucial.

Antidepressant medication can be used to treat poststroke depression, with varying degrees of success. As in all such cases, it is crucial to undertake an accurate assessment of the patient's depression, as the research evidence would suggest that antidepressant medication fails to be an effective treatment for the more mild forms of depression. Not only does antidepressant medication fail to be effective with these more mild presentations, there are also a number of associated negative side effects of taking the medication that are best avoided if at all possible.

Conclusion

Emotional distress following a stroke is extremely common, and for some patients more significant disorders of either depression or anxiety are likely to occur. The presence of emotional distress can have a significant debilitating impact on rehabilitation and recovery. It is therefore important that mood-related problems are correctly assessed and diagnosed, and that effective evidence-based interventions are offered.

Further reading

Barton J. Psychological aspects of stroke. In: (ed.) Kennedy P. *Psychological Management of Physical Disabilities*. London: Routledge, 2007, pp 61–79.

National Institute for Health and Clinical Excellence. Depression in adults with a chronic physical health problem. *Clinical Guideline 91*. London: NICE, 2009.

Royal College of Physicians. *National Clinical Guideline for Stroke*, 3rd edn. London: RCP, 2008.

Thomas SA. Evaluation of anxiety and depression in people with acquired communication impairments. In: (ed.) Brumfitt S. Psychological well-being and acquired communication impairments. Chichester: Wiley-Blackwell, 2009, p 25–43.

CHAPTER 11

Secondary Prevention of Stroke

Duncan Edwards and Jonathan Mant

Addenbrooke's Hospital, University of Cambridge, UK

OVERVIEW

- Patients with stroke or TIA are at high risk of all types of vascular event, not just further stroke
- Current guidelines target 130/80 mmHg for blood pressure reduction
- Statin therapy is indicated after ischaemic stroke or TIA, but should be avoided after haemorrhagic stroke
- Aspirin and dipyridamole are currently recommended for the first two years after ischaemic stroke or TIA
- Patients with atrial fibrillation should be switched from aspirin to warfarin if they experience a first ischaemic stroke or TIA

In the context of stroke and TIA, secondary prevention refers to the prevention of further strokes and vascular events. Modifiable risk factors for stroke should be investigated for all patients in order to design a tailored secondary prevention strategy (Table 11.1). Treatment of all ischaemic strokes, including TIA, incorporates blood pressure lowering, cholesterol lowering, antithrombotic treatment and lifestyle changes. Some specific causes of ischaemic stroke, such as atrial fibrillation and carotid atherosclerosis, merit consideration of further specific measures, such as anticoagulation and carotid endarterectomy. Haemorrhagic stroke requires a different preventive strategy to ischaemic stroke, as antithrombotic treatment and

Table 11.1 Summary of risk factor investigation after stroke/TIA.

Raised blood pressure
Hyperlipidaemia
Diabetes mellitus
Atrial fibrillation and other arrhythmias
Structural cardiac disease
Carotid artery stenosis (only for individuals with a non-disabling carotid territory event likely to benefit from surgery for stenosis)
In any patient where no common cause is identified, fuller investigation for other rare causes should be undertaken by a specialist
Lifestyle factors: smoking; exercise; alcohol; diet

Source: Intercollegiate Stroke Working Party. *National Clinical Guidelines for Stroke*. London: Royal College of Physicians, 2008.

Table 11.2 Quality and Outcomes Framework (QOF) guidance 2009/10.

The practice can produce a register of patients with stroke or TIA (2 points)
The percentage of new patients with stroke or TIA who have been referred for further investigation (2 points)
The percentage of patients with TIA or stroke who have a record of blood pressure in the notes in the preceding 15 months (2 points)
The percentage of patients with a history of TIA or stroke in whom the last blood pressure reading (measured in the previous 15 months) is 150/90 or less (5 points)
The percentage of patients with TIA or stroke who have a record of total cholesterol in the last 15 months (2 points)
The percentage of patients with TIA or stroke whose last measured total cholesterol (measured in the previous 15 months) is 5 mmol/l or less (5 points)
The percentage of patients with a stroke shown to be non-haemorrhagic, or a history of TIA, who have a record that an anti-platelet agent (aspirin, clopidogrel, dipyridamole or a combination) or an anti-coagulant is being taken (unless a contraindication or side effects are recorded (4 points)
The percentage of patients with TIA or stroke who have had influenza immunisation in the preceding 1 September to 31 March (2 points)

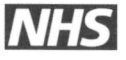

statins may cause more harm than benefit. In the UK, general practices are rewarded for meeting a limited number of secondary prevention quality indicators (Table 11.2).

Risk of recurrence

Patients who have experienced a stroke or a TIA are at high risk of a further vascular event: in a study of patients (mean age 65) with TIA or minor stroke, this risk was shown to be 44% over the ensuing ten years despite aspirin treatment. Risk increases with age and is higher in patients with diabetes. As emphasised in Chapter 3, the risk of recurrent stroke is highest in the first week after the event, and so prompt secondary prevention is vital. A year after the initial stroke or TIA, heart disease is more common than stroke, and so the emphasis of secondary prevention should be on all types of vascular event and not just stroke.

Blood pressure lowering

Historically, clinicians have worried about lowering blood pressure in patients with previous stroke, often due to concerns about efficacy or interfering with the normal physiology of elderly and damaged brains. The PROGRESS trial has refuted this concern and provides good evidence that blood pressure lowering provides substantial benefit in secondary prevention after stroke (Table 11.3). The PROFESS trial also supported this finding, but failed to reach statistical significance, probably because it only achieved a small blood pressure reduction in the treatment group versus the placebo group due to low adherence in the treatment group and high usage of additional antihypertensive agents in the control group (Table 11.4).

The National Clinical Guideline for Stroke currently suggests a target blood pressure of 130/80 for all patients with established cardiovascular disease, including stroke or TIA (Figure 11.1). The one caveat to this target is patients with bilateral, severe (>70%) internal carotid artery stenosis, for whom a target of 150 mmHg systolic is suggested. Choice of therapy is the same as for primary prevention (see Chapter 2).

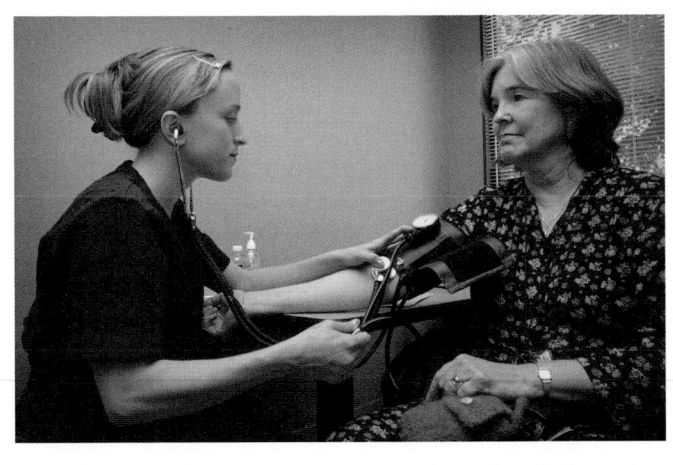

Figure 11.1 Guidelines suggest a blood pressure target in secondary prevention of 130/80. *Source*: James Gathany, National Center for Chronic Disease Prevention and Health.

Cholesterol lowering

It is well established that statins reduce rates of coronary heart disease and major vascular events and this effect has clearly been found in patients with a history of stroke or TIA (Table 11.5). The effect of statins on preventing further stroke is more complex, as statins appear to decrease rates of ischaemic stroke and increase rates of haemorrhagic stroke, and this may account for the failure of some trials to show a significant decrease in all strokes in patients treated with statin therapy. Patients with previous haemorrhagic stroke are more likely to have further haemorrhagic strokes, and for this reason, statins are currently indicated for patients with previous ischaemic stroke or TIA, but should be avoided in patients with previous haemorrhagic stroke unless they have additional cardiac risk factors that outweigh the risk of haemorrhagic stroke. Sub-group analysis of the SPARCL study, in which patients with both haemorrhagic stroke and ischaemic stroke were treated, support this strategy (Figure 11.2).

Table 11.3 Impact of blood pressure-lowering treatment in individuals with previous stroke or TIA, over 4 years.

Outcome	Treatment group (n = 3051)	Placebo group (n = 3054)	Relative risk reduction (95% CI)
Fatal or non-fatal stroke	307	420	28% (17 to 38)
Fatal or disabling stroke	123	181	33% (15 to 46)
Total major vascular events	458	604	26% (16 to 34)
Total deaths	306	319	4% (−12 to 18)

Source: Data from Progress Collaborative Group. Randomised trial of a perindopril-based blood-pressure-lowering regimen among 6,105 individuals with previous stroke or transient ischaemic attack. *Lancet* 2001;**358**(9287): 1033–41.

Table 11.4 The PROGRESS and PROFESS trials.

	PROGRESS	PROFESS
Number of patients in trial	6105 randomised within 5 years after any stroke or TIA	20332 randomised within 90 days after ischaemic stroke
Treatment	Perindopril 4 mg once daily +/− Indapamide 2 mg once daily	Telmisartan 80 mg once daily
Control	Placebo or double placebo	Placebo
Mean follow-up	4 years	2.5 years
Mean excess blood pressure reduction (systolic/diastolic)	9/4 mmHg	3.8/2.0 mmHg
Vascular event relative risk reduction	26% (95% confidence interval 16 to 34)	6% (95% confidence interval −1 to 13)

Source: Data from PROGRESS Collaborative Group. Randomised trial of a perindopril-based blood-pressure-lowering regimen among 6,105 individuals with previous stroke or transient ischaemic attack. *Lancet* 2001;**358**(9287): 1033–41 and Yusuf S, Diener HC, Sacco RL *et al*. Telmisartan to prevent recurrent stroke and cardiovascular events. *N Engl J Med* 2008;**359**(12): 1225–37.

Table 11.5 The Heart Protection and SPARCL trials.

	Heart Protection Study	SPARCL
Number of patients in trial	A prespecified sub-group of 3 280 randomised at least 6 months after ischaemic stroke or TIA	4 731 randomised within 1–6 months after any stroke or TIA
Treatment	Simvastatin 40 mg once daily	Atorvastatin 80 mg once daily
Control	Placebo	Placebo
Mean follow-up	5 years	4.9 years (median)
Vascular event relative risk reduction	20% (95% confidence interval 8 to 29)	20% (95% confidence interval 8 to 31)
Stroke relative risk reduction	2% (95% −21 to 22)	16% (95% confidence interval 1 to 29)

Source: Data from Amarenco P, Bogousslavsky J, Callahan A *et al*. High-dose atorvastatin after stroke or transient ischemic attack. *N Engl J Med* 2006;**355**(6):549–59 and Collins R, Armitage J, Parish S, Sleight P, Peto R. Effects of cholesterol-lowering with simvastatin on stroke and other major vascular events in 20 536 people with cerebrovascular disease or other high-risk conditions. *Lancet* 2004;**363**(9411):757–67.

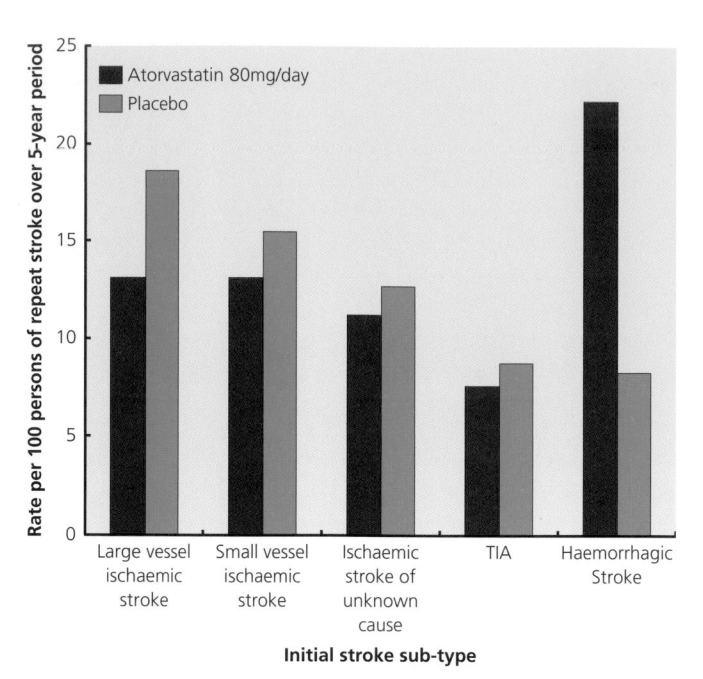

Figure 11.2 Impact of statin therapy on rates of repeat stroke, stratified by initial stroke type.

There is currently little evidence for the use of fibrates in secondary prevention, nor evidence that immediate initiation of statin treatment is superior to late initiation.

NICE currently recommends that for secondary prevention after stroke or TIA, patients should be prescribed 40 mg simvastatin, and medication up-titrated to get total cholesterol below 4 mmol/L and LDL below 2 mmol/L.

Antiplatelet treatment

Unlike in primary prevention, there is clear evidence of a net benefit from aspirin in secondary prevention of serious vascular events. Aspirin reduces serious vascular events by 1.5% per annum and should be started as soon as possible after stroke or TIA. However, aspirin and any antithrombotic therapy increases the risk of bleeding and should be avoided in patients with a previous haemorrhagic stroke unless there is an overwhelming cardiac indication.

The evidence for dual antiplatelet therapy is summarised in Chapter 3, Table 3.3. Dual therapy of dipyridamole and aspirin is the only evidence-based dual antiplatelet therapy available at present, as in the case of other dual antiplatelet strategies the benefit of vascular event reduction is balanced by the harm of increased bleeding (Table 11.6). NICE guidance recommends that a combination of modified-release dipyridamole and aspirin be used in patients who have had an ischaemic stroke or TIA for two years from the most recent event. Dipyridamole is often not tolerated due to headache, in which case aspirin alone should be used. While European and national guidelines permit a dose as low as 50 mg of aspirin for secondary prevention of stroke, the evidence is stronger for a slightly higher dose of 75–150 mg daily for prevention of cardiovascular events.

Table 11.6 Guidance on the use of anti-platelet therapy in secondary prevention.

Aspirin and dipyridamole should be the standard secondary prevention treatment following ischaemic stroke:
- The daily dose of aspirin should be between 50 mg and 300 mg aspirin and dipyridamole MR 200 mg bd
- For patients who are unable to tolerate dipyridamole, aspirin alone is appropriate
- For patients who are intolerant of aspirin, clopidogrel 75 mg once daily is a suitable alternative
- Addition of a proton pump inhibitor should only be considered when there is dyspepsia or other significant risk of gastrointestinal bleeding associated with aspirin, to allow aspirin medication to continue

Source: Intercollegiate Stroke Working Party. *National Clinical Guidelines for Stroke*. London: Royal College of Physicians, 2008.

Lifestyle

Lifestyle measures for secondary prevention are the same as in primary prevention (see Chapter 2 and Figure 11.3). Most of the evidence for these lifestyle measures is extrapolated from primary prevention research; however, since the risk of further events is higher in patients who have already experienced a TIA or stroke, the potential benefits of lifestyle change are greater. Exercise may present particular difficulties due to disability, low fitness or fear of causing harm, and so a tailored programme starting with low-intensity activity and gradually increasing to moderate levels may help.

Observational studies have shown that flu reduces the risk of stroke and so, despite an absence of trial data, the Joint Committee on Vaccination and Immunisations recommends flu vaccination as an effective secondary prevention measure. Hormone replacement therapy and the combined oral contraceptive pill can increase the risk of stroke and should be avoided.

Patient-specific risk factors

Diabetes, atrial fibrillation and structural heart disease should be investigated for and treated if present in all patients with ischaemic

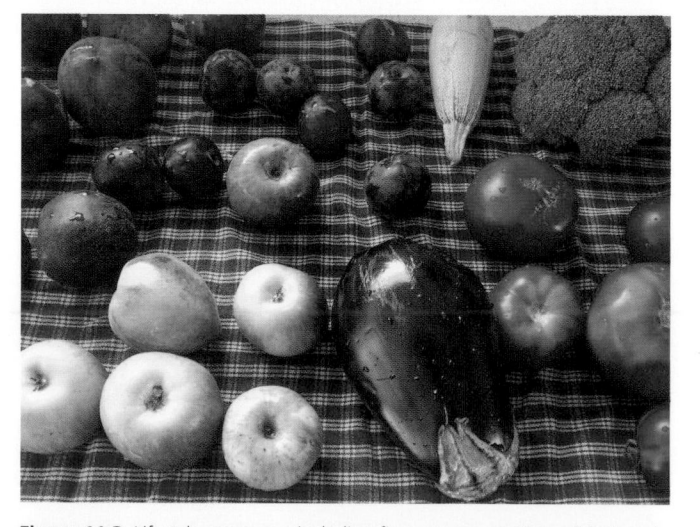

Figure 11.3 Lifestyle measures, including five or more portions of fruit and vegetables per day, are the same as in primary prevention.
Source: Wikimedia Commons.

Table 11.7 Aetiology of stroke in 1 008 consecutive patients aged 15 to 49 with first ever ischaemic stroke.

Aetiology		Number of patients
Cervicocerebral artery dissection		155
Small-vessel disease		139
Large artery atherosclerosis		76
Factor V Leiden mutation		20
Vasculitis		19
Antiphospholipid syndrome		17
SLE		8
Active malignancy		7
Radiation vasculopathy		6
Migrainous infarct		4
Other		26
Undetermined		312
Multiple possible aetiologies		21
Cardioembolism	***Aetiology of cardioembolism***	198
	Dilative cardiomyopathy	33
	Atrial fibrillation	28
	Recent MI (within 1 month)	6
	Congenital cardiac malformation	6
	Infective endocarditis	5
	Mechanical aortic valve	5
	Congestive heart failure	5
	Patent foramen ovale (condition with low or uncertain risk)	87
	Other suspected source	23

Source: Data from Putaala J, Metso AJ, Metso TM *et al*. Analysis of 1008 consecutive patients aged 15 to 49 with first-ever ischemic stroke: The Helsinki young stroke registry. *Stroke* 2009;**40**(4):1195–203.

stroke or TIA. Carotid artery disease should be investigated after any carotid artery territory event, since surgery is indicated if significant carotid artery stenosis is present. A search for rare causes of stroke should only be undertaken when there is a specific clinical suspicion, or in younger patients (usually classified as under the age of 45) with no other identifiable reason for their stroke, under specialist supervision. Cervical artery dissection is a common cause of ischaemic stroke in younger patients (Table 11.7).

Atrial fibrillation

Approximately 15% of ischaemic stroke/TIA patients will also have atrial fibrillation (AF), which may or may not have been previously diagnosed. All undiagnosed patients should be screened by a minimum of a careful history and an ECG. However, AF can be hidden as asymptomatic paroxysmal episodes, which carry a comparable risk of stroke to continuous AF. Strategies to increase diagnostic yield could include regular or opportunistic pulse checks or ECG in general practice, inpatient continuous ECG monitoring, ambulatory ECG monitoring for 24 hours or longer, or an ambulatory ECG event monitor. It is currently unclear what the optimal diagnostic strategy is, but various studies of ambulatory ECG monitoring for between 24 and 72 hours soon after the initial event have resulted in a new diagnosis of AF in between 2.5% and 7.7% of patients screened. Every stroke/TIA patient who is diagnosed with AF or paroxysmal AF should automatically be considered for anticoagulation in preference to aspirin.

Very often patients who are found to require anticoagulation are already taking aspirin for a cardiac indication. The aspirin should be stopped once patients are adequately anticoagulated, as warfarin is as effective as aspirin at preventing myocardial infarction, while the combination of aspirin and anticoagulation presents an unjustified risk of bleeding. Anticoagulation in combination with antiplatelet treatment should only be prescribed in specific high-risk circumstances, such as for patients with prosthetic heart valves, during the first year following percutaneous coronary intervention, and during an episode of acute coronary syndrome.

Structural cardiac disease

Structural cardiac disease can cause thromboembolic stroke. All patients should have a physical examination and ECG, which will not detect all structural cardiac disease. However, an echocardiogram is not essential if the physical examination and ECG are normal and an alternative explanation for the stroke has been found.

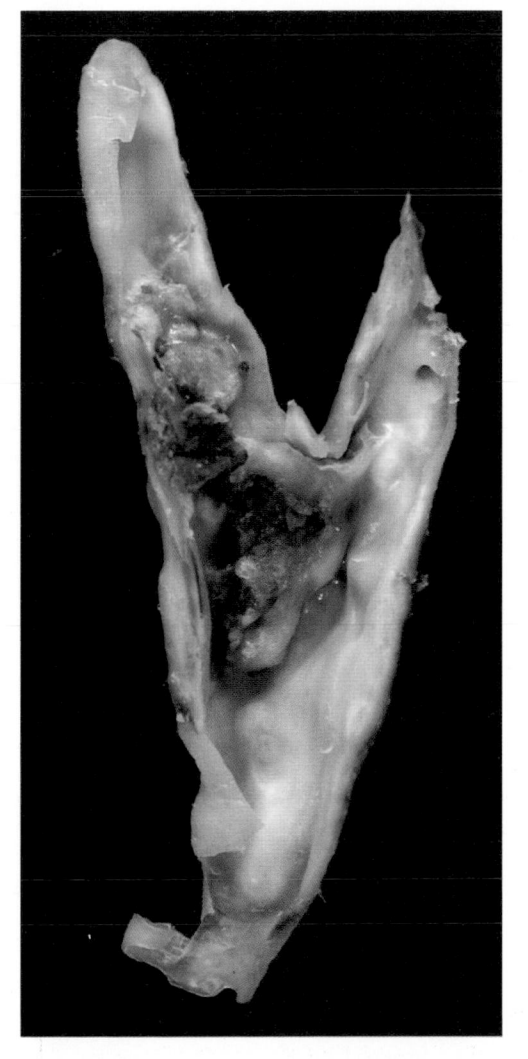

Figure 11.4 The bifurcation of the common carotid artery, with a dark atherosclerotic plaque within the internal carotid artery on the left and the external carotid artery on the right. *Source*: Ed Uthman, MD.

Carotid artery disease

Carotid artery atherosclerosis can result in thromboembolic stroke. This risk of thromboembolism is higher if there is more atherosclerotic plaque, and this is described in terms of stenosis percentage. The risk of thromboembolism is also much higher if a thromboembolism has recently occurred, because the plaque is unstable. Carotid artery disease is treated surgically by endarterectomy, which involves clamping the common carotid, internal carotid and external carotid arteries, then removing the plaque before closing the artery and re-establishing blood flow (Figure 11.4). Carotid endarterectomy carries a risk of perioperative death, stroke and myocardial infarction, which must be carefully balanced against the benefit of stroke prevention.

As described in Chapter 3, earlier treatment of carotid artery disease by carotid endarterectomy provides the most beneficial risk–benefit ratio. Patients with a carotid artery territory stroke/TIA (90% of all ischaemic events) without severe disability should therefore have a non-invasive investigation of the relevant carotid artery, usually carotid duplex ultrasound, performed as quickly as possible. NICE guidelines suggest that carotid endartectomy be performed within two weeks of the initial event in the territory of a carotid artery that has 50–99% stenosis (if the NASCET, North American Symptomatic Carotid Endarterectomy Trial, criteria were used in measurement of stenosis). Patients should have an adequate life expectancy (certainly more than one year) in order for the benefit to fully outweigh the perioperative risk.

Carotid artery stenting carries a doubled risk of perioperative stroke and death versus endarterectomy and is not an alternative outside of clinical trials. For patients who are unfit for endarterectomy, who decline surgery or who do not meet the criteria for surgery, medical therapy and lifestyle measures remain essential and will reduce the risk of thromboembolism.

Further reading

Baigent C, Blackwell L, Collins R *et al.* Aspirin in the primary and secondary prevention of vascular disease: Collaborative meta-analysis of individual participant data from randomised trials. *Lancet* 2009;**373**(9678): 1849–60.

Intercollegiate Stroke Working Party. Chapter 5: Secondary prevention. In: *National Clinical Guidelines for Stroke*. London: Royal College of Physicians, 2008.

Manktelow BN, Potter JF. Interventions in the management of serum lipids for preventing stroke recurrence. *Cochrane Database Syst Rev* 2009;**3**: CD002091.

PROGRESS Collaborative Group. Randomised trial of a perindopril-based blood-pressure-lowering regimen among 6,105 individuals with previous stroke or transient ischaemic attack. *Lancet* 2001;**358**(9287):1033–41.

van Wijk I, Kappelle LJ, van Gijn J *et al.* Long-term survival and vascular event risk after transient ischaemic attack or minor ischaemic stroke: A cohort study. *Lancet* 2005;**365**(9477):2098–104.

CHAPTER 12

Long-term Support for Stroke Survivors and their Carers

Marion F Walker

University of Nottingham, Nottingham, UK

OVERVIEW

- Many stroke survivors have lasting disability and have ongoing rehabilitation and care needs
- Carers require support and help too
- Psychological support is particularly important
- Stroke survivors require periodic review to assess if further input would be beneficial
- Respite care can alleviate the strain of caring
- The benefits of rehabilitation for stroke in care homes is the subject of current research

It is important that acute care is optimised and that stroke survivors receive the best available treatments, such as thrombolysis, in a timely manner. This effective early intervention has been shown to have a positive impact on the reduction of lasting stroke disability and consequently the quality of life of the stroke survivor and their family. The limitation of channelling the majority of health-care efforts and financial resources into the first few hours, days and weeks after stroke is that to date little attention has been paid to the months and years after stroke. This is particularly important as an estimated third of all stroke survivors will have lasting disability. Stroke service audits document that the majority of rehabilitation interventions have been terminated by 3–6 months after stroke and, indeed, experts have previously rationalised that all stroke survivors had reached a plateau in their recovery by this time period.

Sadly, it is well documented that when stroke services finally withdraw from active intervention, stroke survivors and their carers report feeling isolated and abandoned, yet many still experience lasting disability. From the available stroke literature, we are aware that some stroke survivors can still make a tangible recovery months and years after stroke. While the burden of caring for a disabled individual has been widely recognised by the stroke community, little is done to actively provide ongoing physical and psychological support to carers. It is therefore important to insure that stroke survivors and their carers can, and know how to, gain access to rehabilitation and support services when required regardless of the time interval since the stroke onset.

Assessment of ongoing stroke needs

The National Stroke Strategy has recommended that all patients receive rehabilitation and support for as long as required. It also recommends that every stroke survivor has a six-month and annual follow-up to identify if further rehabilitative input is required (Figure 12.1).

But what components should this assessment contain, what services are available to access once the assessment has been completed and, indeed, who should conduct this assessment? These questions

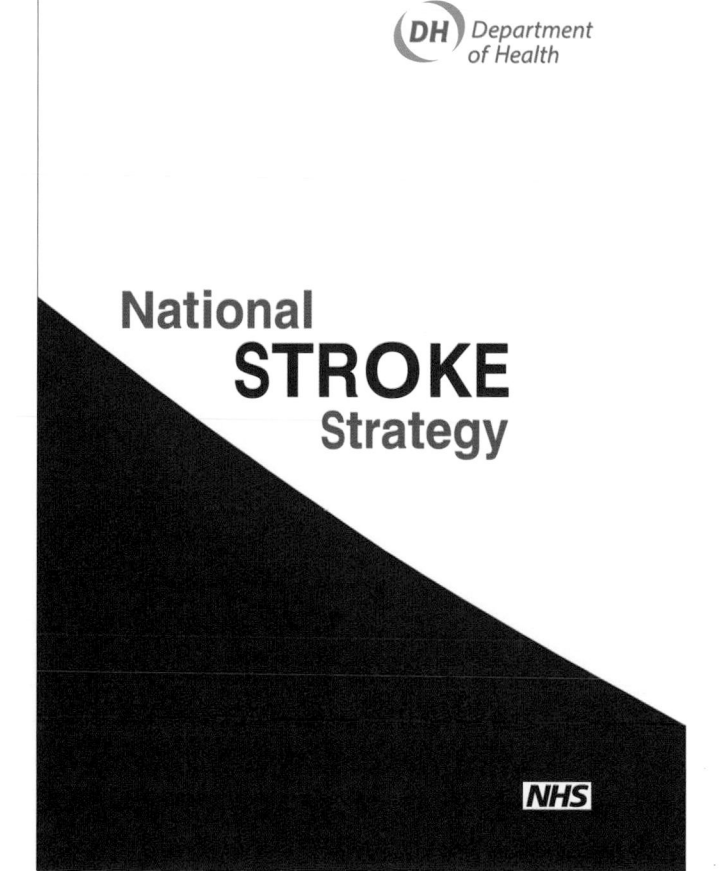

Figure 12.1 National Stroke Strategy.

ABC of Stroke. Edited by Jonathan Mant and Marion F Walker.
© 2011 Blackwell Publishing Ltd.

49

are currently being addressed in each geographical location, as available services and workforce mobilisation issues are so varied across the UK. In the current economic climate it may be necessary for the stroke community to reconfigure existing services and optimise the use of the relevant voluntary organisations, as it is unlikely that new money will be available to commission new long-term stroke services. The third sector, such as the services provided by the Stroke Association, is likely to be in greater demand as stroke-care providers endeavour to meet the ongoing needs of those affected by stroke.

To meet these needs it will be important that all health, physical, psychological, and social care needs are addressed during any follow-up stroke assessment, and this will obviously necessitate joint working between health and social care. In particular, it is very important that stroke survivors have access to services providing psychological support, as this requirement is not always immediately identified or required in the early stages of the stroke journey.

The role of the third sector in long-term care

The Stroke Association is the main stroke charity in the UK and is of tremendous value to all those affected by stroke as they come to terms with their new life in the months and years that follow. One of the charity's key roles is to provide information to stroke survivors, their family and their carers. The Stroke Association website (www.stroke.org.uk) provides a wealth of practical information, with downloadable fact sheets to assist the individual in their quest for information. Leaflets, fact sheets and resource sheets are available on a wide range of topics, including how to source benefits, sex after stroke, rehabilitation, driving after stroke, taste changes after stroke and private treatment, to name but a few (see Figures 12.2, 12.3 and 12.4). The Stroke Association also provide a wealth of services in the community to assist those who live with the long-term consequences of stroke, such as long-term support groups, life after stroke services, communication support coordinators, family and carer support coordinators and stroke clubs. Information is provided on the services available in each geographical area in the UK, with contact numbers readily available. A TalkStroke messaging forum is also available via the website, where survivors and their carers can post questions, tell their own story and provide and receive peer support. Such services are invaluable to individuals who still require support.

While ongoing information gathering is important for patients and their relatives, research available on this topic would suggest that different levels of information are required at different times in the aftermath of stroke and that this may vary from patient to patient. A recent Cochrane Systematic review on information giving to stroke patients indicated that the best way to provide information is in a structured learning environment, not by giving leaflets alone.

The long-term psychological and physical demands made on carers can have a devastating impact on marital and family relationships and also on the health of the carer. Long-term support in terms of respite care for carers can be accessed through other voluntary organisations such as Crossroads Care (www.crossroads.org.uk).

Crossroads Care provides support and care for individuals whose carers need a break away from their loved ones. It is a national network with over 5000 trained carers. It is a national registered charity and is a not-for-profit organisation. There are various funding schemes available and services may be paid for directly via the individual's local authority or through self-funding methods.

Vitalise (www.vitalise.org.uk) is another well-resourced organisation that provides a variety of services for individuals and their carers requiring a break away from home. Included in the services offered are short respite breaks, accessible adventure activity breaks, self-catering lodges and long-stay services. Four Vitalise centres are available in the UK and 24-hour nursing care and personal support can be provided if required.

Leisure and social reintegration

Reintegration into the community after stroke provides tangible evidence of the restoration of a prestroke lifestyle. This in turn can have a major effect in lifting the self-esteem and mood of the individual. For many people a visit to the cinema, theatre, evening class or outing to the local pub is just as an important part of life after a stroke as it was prior to the onset of stroke. Despite this desire, many people require a lot of support to return to such activities, even those who have made an excellent recovery, as self-confidence may have been lost.

For survivors with physical impairments, ramps, wheelchair access and disabled toilets are now thankfully part of most public buildings. Many stroke survivors can return to hobbies that have given a lifetime of pleasure, such as playing chess, computer games, painting, building model aeroplanes, bird watching, furniture restoration, reading, dancing and so on (Figure 12.5). However, many have such severe physical or cognitive impairments that this may no longer be possible. If adaptations cannot be made to the activity itself or the equipment used, then an alternative hobby or interest should be found. Great consideration should be given to the benefits that the previous hobby offered so that similar challenges or rewards can be achieved from the new interest.

In some circumstances stroke survivors do not return to previous leisure pursuits, not because they physically or psychologically cannot take part, but simply due to transport difficulties. In such circumstances, information on Dial-a-ride or voluntary driving schemes should be offered. Stroke survivors will usually require an able-bodied friend or relative to accompany them on their first few journeys as they build up their confidence in using such services. Drivers operating in these schemes are trained to deal with a variety of physical disabilities and will provide reassurance that this is a method of transport that will deal with the individual's physical limitations in a sensitive manner.

Environmental adaptations

Initially on returning home from hospital many stroke survivors will temporarily adjust their living arrangements to suit their disability while their confidence grows. For some that may mean going to live with a family member for a short period of time, for others it may mean converting a dining room or living room on the ground

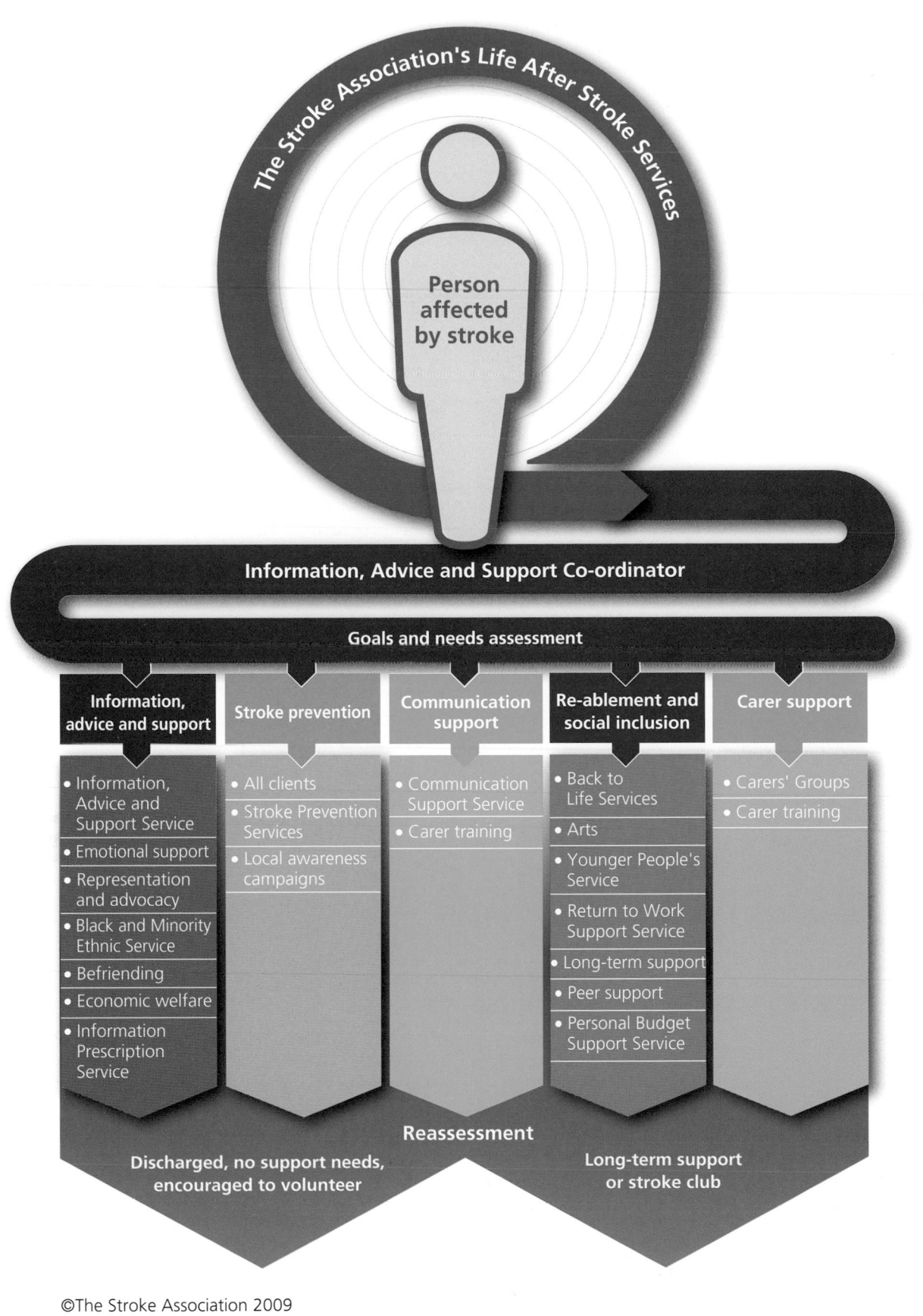

©The Stroke Association 2009

Figure 12.2 TSA Life after stroke model.

floor of their home into a temporary bedroom, with commode or other toilet facilities. If it becomes apparent that this is no longer a temporary solution, the local authority occupational therapist may become involved and will assess the home environment for adaptations for independent living. Such adaptations may include

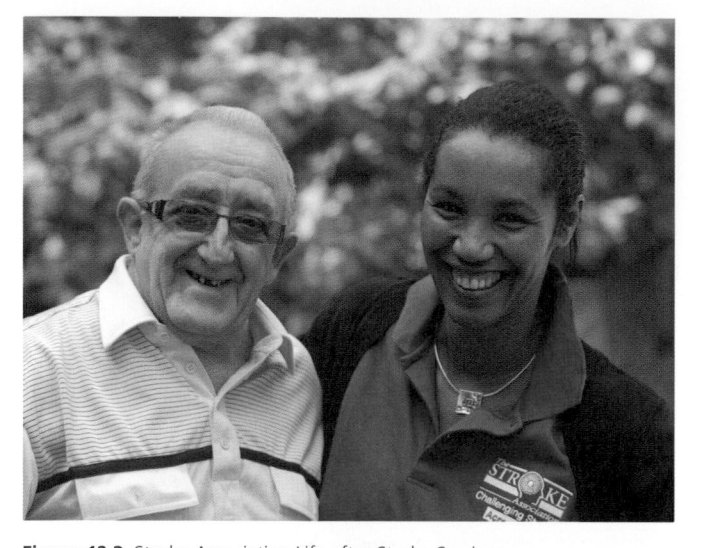

Figure 12.3 Stroke Association Life after Stroke Services.

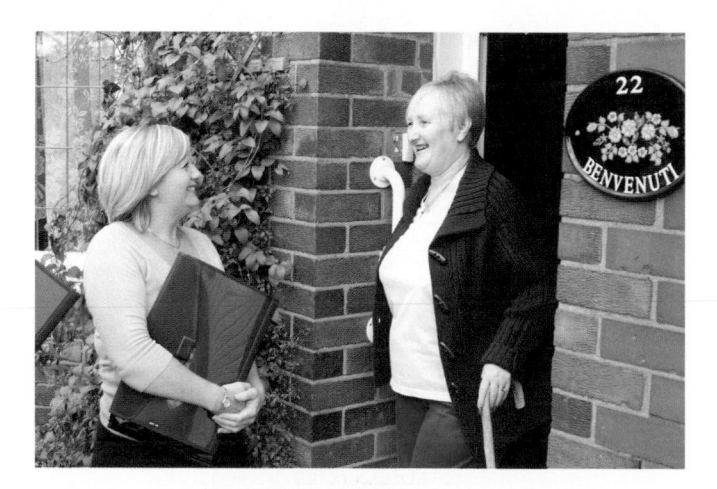

Figure 12.4 Supporting life after stroke.

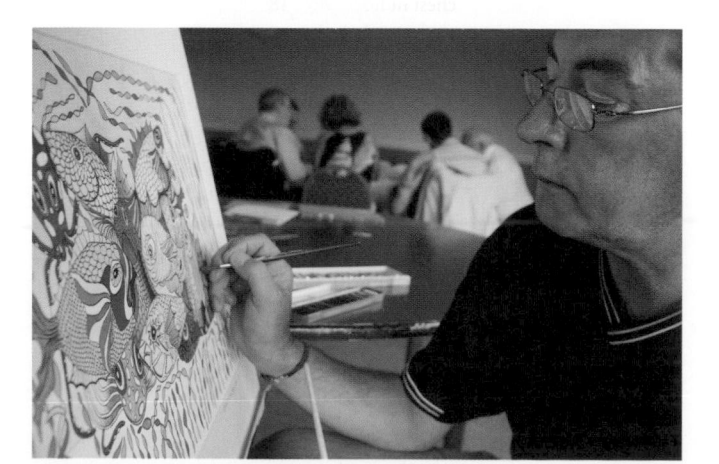

Figure 12.5 Leisure after stroke.

second stair rails to allow safe access to upper floors, adapted toilets and bathrooms, ramps for wheelchair access, through-ceiling lifts or stair lifts. Smaller pieces of equipment may also be provided, such as bathing or showering equipment or appliances to assist in feeding and dressing. Equipment can be purchased or provided on short- or long-term loan and grants can be obtained for major structural work. Referrals to local authority occupational therapists can be made by the general practitioner or directly by the family themselves.

Rehabilitation in care homes

Admission to specialised multi-disciplinary stroke units not only reduces the odds of death and disability, but also those of being admitted to a nursing or residential care home. Yet despite this reduction, 17% of hospital discharges are to care homes. This population consequently have more severe impairments and activity limitations than those who return home, with 65% experiencing cognitive impairments, 40% mood disorders and 75% incontinence. Such problems have a great impact on a resident's ability to carry out the self-care activities of daily living and can have a significant effect on mobility.

National surveys have described a lack of rehabilitation provision in care homes, with as few as 3% of care home residents accessing therapy services. This is in direct contrast to other countries, where provision is reported to be high. Evidence for the efficacy of rehabilitation input to care homes is, however, conflicting and confusing, and more research is needed in this area to establish the effectiveness and cost effectiveness of rehabilitation input. Nevertheless, there is some evidence from the UK to support the provision of occupational therapy for stroke residents, with a reduction in deterioration in self-care tasks and mobility compared to those residents who didn't receive this service. The rehabilitation input in this study incorporated interventions to improve independence in toileting, feeding, mobility and dressing, and gave particular attention to addressing environmental barriers such as ensuring bed and chair heights were at an appropriate height, grab handles and toilet frames were in situ to ensure independence and mobility aids were appropriately prescribed and well maintained. A large multi-centre trial called the Occupational Therapy in Care Home (OTCH) study, funded by the Health Technology Assessment, is now underway, reporting in 2014, and this will provide definitive evidence on the benefits of occupational therapy provision in care homes.

Further reading

Aziz NA, Leonardi-Bee J, Phillips MF, Gladman J, Legg LA, Walker MF. Therapy-based rehabilitation services for patients living at home more than one year after stroke. *Cochrane Database of Systematic Reviews* 2008, Issue 2.

Department of Health. *National Stroke Strategy.* London: Department of Health Publications, 2007.

Sackley CM, Copley Atkinson J, Walker MF. Occupational therapy in nursing and residential care settings: A description of a randomised controlled trial intervention. *British Journal of Occupational Therapy* 2004;**6**(73):104–10.

Smith J, Forster A, House A, Knapp P, Wright JJ, Young J. Information provision for stroke patients and their caregivers. *Cochrane Database of Systematic Reviews* 2008, Issue 2.

Index

CURRENT TITLES

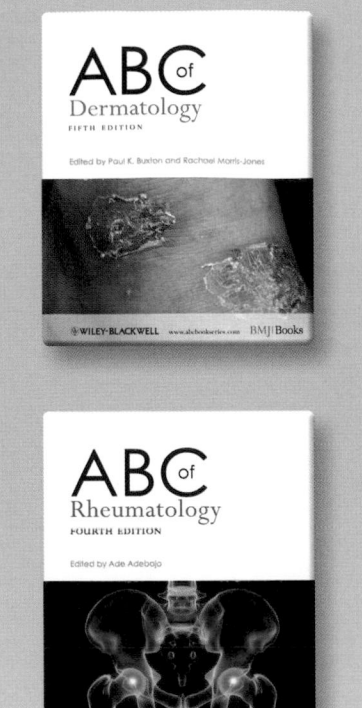

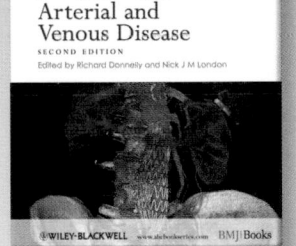

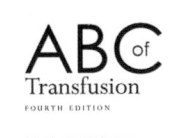

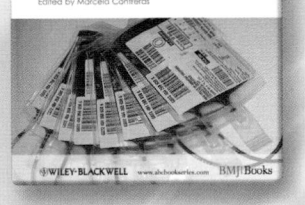

ABC of Dermatology
5TH EDITION

**Edited by Paul K. Buxton &
Rachael Morris-Jones**
Consultant Dermatologist, Hampshire;
King's College Hospital, London

- A new 20th anniversary edition of this
  bestselling *ABC* covering the diagnosis and
  treatment of skin conditions for the non-
  dermatologist
- Covers the core knowledge on therapy,
  management and diagnosis of common
  conditions and highlights the evidence
  base
- Provides clear learning outcomes and basic
  science boxes
- Includes a new chapter on the general
  principles of skin condition management
  for specialist nurses

**March 2009 | 9781405170659 | 224 pages
£28.99/US$52.95/€35.90/AU$57.95**

ABC of Rheumatology
4TH EDITION

Edited by Ade Adebajo
University of Sheffield

- A practical guide to the diagnosis and
  treatment of rheumatology for the non-
  specialist
- Fully revised and updated to include
  information on new treatments and
  therapies while covering the core
  knowledge on therapy, management and
  diagnosis
- A highly illustrated, informative and
  practical source of knowledge offering links
  to further information and resources
- This established *ABC* is an accessible
  reference for all primary care health
  professionals

**October 2009 | 9781405170680 | 192 pages
£27.99/US$44.95/€34.90/AU$57.95**

ABC of Arterial and Venous Disease
2ND EDITION

**Edited by Richard Donnelly &
Nick J.M. London**
University of Nottingham;
University of Leicester

- A practical guide to the diagnosis and
  treatment of arterial and venous disease for
  the non-specialist, focusing on the modern
  day management of patients
- Explains the different interventions for
  arterial and venous disease
- Covers the core knowledge on therapy,
  management and diagnosis and highlights
  the evidence base on varicose veins,
  diabetes, blood clots, stroke and TIA and
  use of stents
- This revised new edition now includes
  information on new treatments and
  therapies, antithrombotic therapy, and non-
  invasive techniques

**April 2009 | 9781405178891 | 120 pages
£26.99/US$49.95/€33.90/AU$54.95**

ABC of Transfusion
4TH EDITION

Edited by Marcela Contreras
Royal Free and University College Hospitals
Medical School, London

- A comprehensive and highly regarded
  guide to all the practical aspects of blood
  transfusion
- This new edition is an established reference
  from a leading centre in transfusion
- Includes five new chapters on variant CJD,
  stem cell transplantation, immunotherapy,
  blood matching and appropriate use of
  transfusion
- Reflects the latest developments in blood
  transfusion management

**March 2009 | 9781405156462 | 128 pages
£26.99/US$49.95/€33.90/AU$54.95**

For more information on any of the titles, please visit the *ABC* website at **www.abcbookseries.com**

CURRENT TITLES

ABC of Mental Health
2ND EDITION

Edited by Teifion Davies & Tom Craig
Both King's College, London Institute of Psychiatry

- Provides clear practical advice on how to recognise, diagnose and manage mental disorders successfully and safely

- Includes sections on selecting drugs and psychological treatments, and improving compliance

- Contains information on the major categories of mental health disorders, the mental health needs of vulnerable groups (such as the elderly, children, homeless and ethnic minorities) and psychological treatments

- Covers the mental health needs of special groups: equips GPs and hospital doctors with all the information they need for the day to day management of patients with mental health problems

**May 2009 | 9780727916396 | 128 pages
£27.99/US$47.95/€34.90/AU$57.95**

ABC of Lung Cancer

Edited by Ian Hunt, Martin M. Muers & Tom Treasure
Guy's Hospital, London; Leeds General Infirmary; Guy's & St. Thomas' Hospital, London

- A practical guide for those involved in the care of the lung cancer patient

- An up-to-date evidence-based review of one of the most common cancers in the western world

- Written by the specialists involved in the launch of the NICE UK Lung Cancer Guidelines

- Looks at the epidemiology and diagnosis of lung cancer, focusing particularly on primary care issues

**April 2009 | 9781405146524 | 64 pages
£21.99/US$37.95/€27.90/AU$44.95**

ABC of Spinal Disorders

Edited by Andrew Clarke, Alwyn Jones, Michael O'Malley & Robert McLaren
Royal Devon and Exeter Hospital; University of Wales Hospital, Cardiff; Warrington Hospital; GP

- This brand new title addresses the causes and management of the different spinal conditions presenting in general practice

- Provides much needed practical guidance on the diagnosis, treatment and advice as back pain is one of the commonest causes for absence from work and is a chronic problem confronting general practitioners

- Includes guidance for the GP when they have to refer patients for more specialist treatment

**December 2009 | 9781405170697 | 72 pages
£19.99/US$35.95/€24.90/AU$39.95**

ABC of Medical Law

Lorraine Corfield, Ingrid Granne & William Latimer-Sayer
Guy's and St Thomas' NHS Trust, London; University of Oxford; Lawyer, Clinical Negligence and Personal Injury Specialist

- Fills the gap for a basic introduction to legal issues in health care that is easy to understand and act upon

- Provides up to date coverage of contentious issues such as withholding and withdrawing treatment and confidentiality

- Accessible to those without any legal knowledge, providing guidance without becoming embroiled in complicated legal discussion

**June 2009 | 9781405176286 | 64 pages
£19.99/US$35.95/€24.90/AU$39.95**

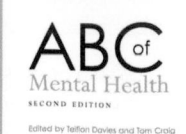
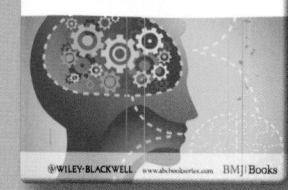
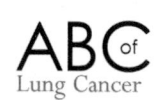
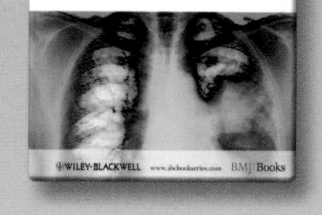
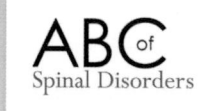
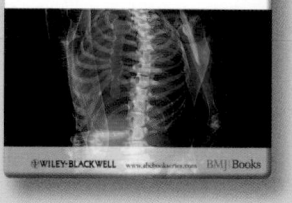
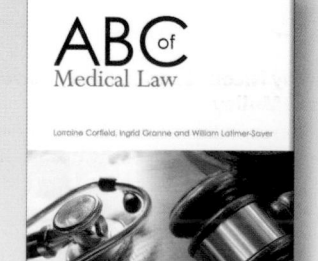

CURRENT TITLES

ABC of the First Year
6TH EDITION

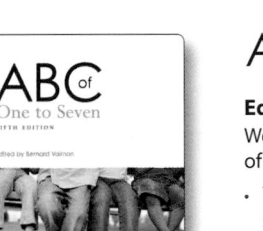

Bernard Valman & Roslyn Thomas
Both Northwick Park Hospital, Harrow, Middlesex

- Includes new sections on recognition and prevention of obesity in weaning, and good weaning practices
- Helps practitioners answer parents and carers questions about what's normal and what's a concern
- Includes a Development Chart (up to 2 years of age) showing the normal range and different cut-offs, in different abilities or activities
- Features recommendations that conform to the latest NICE guidelines
- Includes useful links and addresses such as patient resources and organisations

January 2009 | 9781405180375 | 136 pages | £26.99/US$49.95/€33.90/AU$54.95

ABC of One to Seven
5TH EDITION

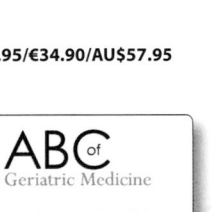

Edited by Bernard Valman
Northwick Park Hospital, Harrow, Middlesex

- Provides a guide to the diseases, developmental disorders, and emotional problems of early childhood
- Each chapter contains concise advice on the child health problems most frequently encountered by primary health care workers
- Includes new chapters on prevention and management of obesity, immunisation, and a section on ADHD and autism with guidance on what to refer and when, and how to manage afterwards
- Includes a Development Chart, covering the full age range, showing the normal range and different cut-offs, in different abilities and activities
- Includes an appendix of patient resources including links to organisations, the department of health and the Royal Colleges, and a chapter explaining NHS direct and changes to legislation for social services following the Children Act

October 2009 | 9781405181051 | 168 pages | £27.99/US$47.95/€34.90/AU$57.95

ABC of Geriatric Medicine

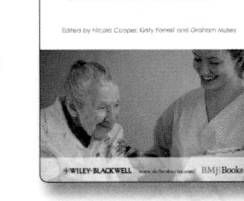

Edited by Nicola Cooper, Kirsty Forrest & Graham Mulley
Leeds General Infirmary; Leeds Teaching Hospital NHS Trust; St James's University Hospital, Leeds

- A practical guide for all who care for older people
- Provides an overview of key topics in geriatric medicine with references, further reading and resources
- Based on the UK specialty training curriculum in geriatric medicine

January 2009 | 9781405169424 | 88 pages | £21.99/US$39.95/€27.90/AU$44.95

ABC of Emergency Differential Diagnosis

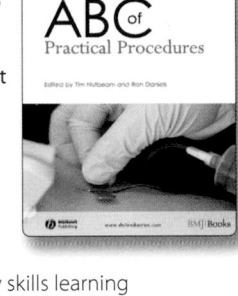

Edited by Francis Morris & Alan Fletcher
Both Northern General Hospital, Sheffield

- A practical, step-by-step guide to the diagnosis and treatment of acute conditions for non-specialists
- Covers the essentials on symptoms, assessment, diagnosis, treatment and management of the most important conditions
- Includes 'walk-through' diagnosis, clear learning outcomes, and easy to find treatment options
- Takes a problem-based approach for the rapid assimilation of information
- Features case studies that allow the reader to be sure that they have synthesised the information given and can apply it to clinical cases

July 2009 | 9781405170635 | 96 pages | £26.99/US$49.95/€32.90/AU$54.95

ABC of Practical Procedures

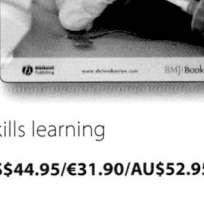

Edited by Tim Nutbeam & Ron Daniels
West Midlands Deanery; Good Hope Hospital, Heart of England Foundation Trust, Birmingham

- Teaches the core skills required of all doctors in training
- Features each stage of each procedure in colour step-by-step photographs as it is being performed
- Features a useful tips/handy hints box to aid key skills learning

November 2009 | 9781405185950 | 144 pages | £25.99/US$44.95/€31.90/AU$52.95

ABC of Sepsis

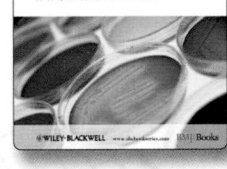

Edited by Ron Daniels & Tim Nutbeam
Good Hope Hospital, Heart of England Foundation Trust, Birmingham, Surviving Sepsis Campaign UK and Survive Sepsis; West Midlands Deanery and Survive Sepsis

- A much needed introduction to this important subject - a core aspect of acute medicine in the UK
- Offers a basic introduction to sepsis for trainees and the MDT
- A timely subject due to current concerns regarding hospital infection and patient safety
- The authors are involved with the Surviving Sepsis campaign, developed to improve the management, diagnosis and treatment of sepsis

December 2009 | 9781405181945 | 104 pages | £25.99/US$46.95/€32.90/AU$52.95

ALSO AVAILABLE

ABC of Adolescence
Russell Viner
2005 | 9780727915740 | 56 pages | £22.99/US$37.95/€28.90/AU$47.95

ABC of Allergies
Stephen R. Durham
1998 | 9780727912367 | 65 pages | £25.99/US$47.95/€32.90/AU$52.95

ABC of Antenatal Care, 4th Edition
Geoffrey Chamberlain & Margery Morgan
2002 | 9780727916921 | 92 pages | £23.99/US$44.95/€29.90/AU$47.95

ABC of Antithrombotic Therapy
Gregory Y.H. Lip & Andrew D. Blann
2003 | 9780727917713 | 67 pages | £21.99/US$37.95/€27.90/AU$44.95

ABC of Brain Stem Death, 2nd Edition
Christopher Pallis & D.H. Harley
1996 | 9780727902450 | 55 pages | £26.99/US$49.95/€32.90/AU$54.95

ABC of Breast Diseases, 3rd Edition
J. Michael Dixon
2005 | 9780727918284 | 120 pages | £28.99/US$53.95/€35.90/AU$57.95

ABC of Burns
Shehan Hettiaratchy, Remo Papini & Peter Dziewulski
2004 | 9780727917874 | 56 pages | £21.99/US$37.95/€27.90/AU$44.95

ABC of Child Protection, 4th Edition
Sir Roy Meadow, Jacqueline Mok & Donna Rosenberg
2007 | 9780727918178 | 120 pages | £28.99/US$53.95/€34.90/AU$57.95

ABC of Clinical Electrocardiography, 2nd Edition
Francis Morris, William Brady & John Camm
2008 | 9781405170642 | 112 pages | £27.99/US$52.95/€34.90/AU$57.95

ABC of Clinical Genetics, 3rd Edition
Helen M. Kingston
2002 | 9780727916273 | 120 pages | £26.99/US$50.95/€33.90/AU$54.95

ABC of Clinical Haematology, 3rd Edition
Drew Provan
2007 | 9781405153539 | 112 pages | £28.99/US$53.95/€35.90/AU$57.95

ABC of Colorectal Diseases, 2nd Edition
David Jones
1998 | 9780727911056 | 110 pages | £28.99/US$53.95/€34.90/AU$57.95

ABC of Complementary Medicine, 2nd Edition
Catherine Zollman, Andrew Vickers & Janet Richardson
2008 | 9781405136570 | 58 pages | £22.99/US$42.95/€28.90/AU$47.95

ABC of Conflict and Disaster
Anthony Redmond, Peter F. Mahoney, James Ryan, Cara Macnab & Lord David Owen
2005 | 9780727917263 | 80 pages | £21.99/US$37.95/€27.90/AU$44.95

ABC of COPD
Graeme P. Currie
2006 | 9781405147118 | 48 pages | £21.99/US$37.95/€27.90/AU$44.95

ABC of Ear, Nose and Throat, 5th Edition
Harold S. Ludman & Patrick Bradley
2007 | 9781405136563 | 120 pages | £28.99/US$53.95/€35.90/AU$57.95

ABC of Eating Disorders
Jane Morris
2008 | 9780727918437 | 80 pages | £21.99/US$37.95/€27.90/AU$44.95

ABC of Emergency Radiology, 2nd Edition
Otto Chan
2007 | 9780727915283 | 144 pages | £29.99/US$53.95/€36.90/AU$59.95

ABC of Eyes, 4th Edition
Peng T. Khaw, Peter Shah & Andrew R. Elkington
2004 | 9780727916594 | 104 pages | £27.99/US$49.95/€34.90/AU$57.95

ABC of Headache
Anne MacGregor & Alison Frith
2008 | 9781405170666 | 88 pages | £21.99/US$37.95/€27.90/AU$44.95

ABC of Health Informatics
Frank Sullivan & Jeremy Wyatt
2006 | 9780727918505 | 56 pages | £21.99/US$37.95/€27.90/AU$44.95

ABC of Heart Failure, 2nd Edition
Russell C. Davis, Michael K. Davies & Gregory Y.H. Lip
2006 | 9780727916440 | 72 pages | £21.99/US$37.95/€27.90/AU$44.95

ABC of Hypertension, 5th Edition
Gareth Beevers, Gregory Y.H. Lip & Eoin O'Brien
2007 | 9781405130615 | 88 pages | £26.99/US$47.95/€32.90/AU$54.95

ABC of Interventional Cardiology
Ever D. Grech
2003 | 9780727915467 | 51 pages | £21.99/US$37.95/€27.90/AU$44.95

ABC of Kidney Disease
David Goldsmith, Satishkumar Abeythunge Jayawardene & Penny Ackland
2007 | 9781405136754 | 96 pages | £27.99/US$52.95/€34.90/AU$57.95

ABC of Labour Care
Geoffrey Chamberlain, Philip Steer & Luke Zander
1999 | 9780727914156 | 60 pages | £19.99/US$35.95/€24.90/AU$39.95

ABC of Liver, Pancreas and Gall Bladder
Ian Beckingham
2001 | 9780727915313 | 64 pages | £19.99/US$35.95/€24.90/AU$39.95

ABC of Major Trauma, 3rd Edition
Peter Driscoll, David Skinner & Richard Earlam
1999 | 9780727913784 | 192 pages | £25.99/US$49.95/€31.90/AU$52.95

ABC of Monitoring Drug Therapy
Jeffrey Aronson, M. Hardman & D.J.M. Reynolds
1993 | 9780727907912 | 46 pages | £21.99/US$37.95/€27.90/AU$44.95

ABC of Nutrition, 4th Edition
A. Stewart Truswell
2003 | 9780727916648 | 152 pages | £26.99/US$49.95/€32.90/AU$54.95

ABC of Obesity
Naveed Sattar & Mike Lean
2007 | 9781405136747 | 64 pages | £21.99/US$35.95/€27.90/AU$44.95

ABC of Occupational and Environmental Medicine, 2nd Edition
David Snashall & Dipti Patel
2003 | 9780727916112 | 124 pages | £28.99/US$53.95/€35.90/AU$57.95

ABC of Oral Health
Crispian Scully
2000 | 9780727915511 | 41 pages | £19.99/US$35.95/€24.90/AU$39.95

ABC of Palliative Care, 2nd Edition
Marie Fallon & Geoffrey Hanks
2006 | 9781405130790 | 96 pages | £24.99/US$47.95/€30.90/AU$49.95

ABC of Patient Safety
John Sandars & Gary Cook
2007 | 9781405156929 | 64 pages | £23.99/US$42.95/€29.90/AU$47.95

ABC of Preterm Birth
William McGuire & Peter Fowlie
2005 | 9780727917638 | 56 pages | £21.99/US$37.95/€27.90/AU$44.95

ABC of Psychological Medicine
Richard Mayou, Michael Sharpe & Alan Carson
2003 | 9780727915566 | 72 pages | £22.99/US$37.95/€27.90/AU$47.95

ABC of Resuscitation, 5th Edition
Michael Colquhoun, Anthony Handley & T.R. Evans
2003 | 9780727916693 | 111 pages | £28.99/US$53.95/€34.90/AU$57.95

ABC of Sexual Health, 2nd Edition
John Tomlinson
2004 | 9780727917591 | 96 pages | £25.99/US$47.95/€32.90/AU$52.95

ABC of Sexually Transmitted Infections, 5th Edition
Michael W. Adler, Frances Cowan, Patrick French, Helen Mitchell & John Richens
2004 | 9780727917614 | 104 pages | £25.99/US$49.95/€31.90/AU$52.95

ABC of Skin Cancer
Sajjad Rajpar & Jerry Marsden
2008 | 9781405162197 | 80 pages | £21.99/US$41.95/€27.90/AU$44.95

ABC of Smoking Cessation
John Britton
2004 | 9780727918185 | 56 pages | £18.99/US$35.95/€22.90/AU$37.95

ABC of Sports and Exercise Medicine, 3rd Edition
Gregory Whyte, Mark Harries & Clyde Williams
2005 | 9780727918130 | 136 pages | £28.99/US$56.95/€34.90/AU$57.95

ABC of Subfertility
Peter Braude & Alison Taylor
2004 | 9780727915344 | 64 pages | £19.99/US$35.95/€24.90/AU$39.95

ABC of Tubes, Drains, Lines and Frames
Adam Brooks, Peter F. Mahoney & Brian Rowlands
2008 | 9781405160148 | 88 pages | £21.99/US$37.95/€27.90/AU$44.95

ABC of the Upper Gastrointestinal Tract
Robert Logan, Adam Harris, J.J. Misiewicz & J.H. Baron
2002 | 9780727912664 | 54 pages | £21.99/US$37.95/€27.90/AU$44.95

ABC of Urology, 2nd Edition
Chris Dawson & Hugh N. Whitfield
2006 | 9781405139595 | 64 pages | £22.99/US$42.95/€27.90/AU$47.95

ABC of Wound Healing
Joseph E. Grey & Keith G. Harding
2006 | 9780727916952 | 56 pages | £21.99/US$37.95/€27.90/AU$44.95